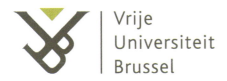 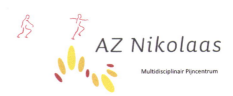

Faculteit Geneeskunde en Farmacie

Direct and Indirect Ganglion Stimulation for the Management of Chronic Pain.

Insights, Techniques and Results

Proefschrift voorgelegd met het oog op het behalen van de graad van
Doctor in de Medische wetenschappen aan de
Vrije Universiteit Brussel
Te verdedigen door

Jean Pierre Van Buyten

Promotor	Prof. dr. Maarten Moens	UZ Brussel, Dienst Neurochirurgie en Radiologie, Brussel, België
Co-promotores	Prof. dr. Koen Paemeleire	UZ Gent, Dienst Neurologie, Gent, België
	Prof. dr. Frank Huygen	Erasmus MC, Dienst Anesthesiologie en Pijn Centrum, Rotterdam, Nederland

Print: Silhouet, Maldegem

© 2017 Jean Pierre Van Buyten
© 2017 Uitgeverij VUBPRESS Brussels University Press
VUBPRESS is an imprint of ASP nv (Academic and Scientific Publishers nv)
Keizerslaan 34
B-1000 Brussels
Tel. +32 (0)2 289 26 56
Fax +32 (0)2 289 26 59
E-mail: info@vubpress.be
www.vubpress.be

Cover photo: Marc Nollet

ISBN 978 90 5718 647 9
NUR 870
Legal deposit D/2017/11.161/038

All rights reserved. No parts of this book may be reproduced or transmitted in any form or by any means, electronic, mechanical, photocopying, recording, or otherwise, without the prior written permission of the author.

First, they ignore you,
then they laugh at you,
then they fight you,
then you win.

Mahatma Gandhi

Leden van de examencommissie

Prof. dr. Jan Lamote (voorzitter)
Dienst Heelkunde.
Universitair Ziekenhuis Brussel

Prof. dr. Erik Cattrysse
Dienst Experimentele Anatomie (EXAN), vakgroep Kinesitherapie, Menselijke Fysiologie en Anatomie (KIMA)
Vrije Universiteit Brussel

Prof. dr. Ann De Smedt
Dienst Neurologie, en dienst Fysische Geneeskunde en Revalidatie
Universitair Ziekenhuis Brussel

Prof. dr. Jacques Devulder
Dienst Anesthesiologie en Multidisciplinair Pijncentrum
Universitair Ziekenhuis, Gent

Prof. dr. Maarten van Kleef
Dienst Anesthesiologie en Pijn centrum
Maastricht Universitair Medisch Centrum, Maastricht, Nederland

Dit manuscript voor het behalen van de titel
philosophiae doctor (PhD) in de medische wetenschappen
is gebaseerd op:

Chronic stimulation of the Gasserian ganglion in patients with trigeminal neuropathy: A case series.
Van Buyten JP, Hens C.
J of Neurosurgical review. 2011;1:73-77

Electromagnetic Navigation Technology for More Precise Electrode Placement in the Foramen Ovale: A Technical Report
Van Buyten J, Smet I, Van de Kelft E.
Neuromodulation. 2009;12:244-249.

Stimulation of the Gasserian ganglion in the treatment of refractory trigeminal neuropathy.
Kustermans L, Van Buyten JP, Smet I, Coucke W, Politis C.
J Craniomaxillofac Surg. 2017;45:39-46.

Phenotype of patients responsive to occipital nerve stimulation for refractory head pain.
Paemeleire K, Van Buyten JP, Van Buynder M, Alicino D, Van Maele G, Smet I, Goadsby P. J.
Cephalalgia. 2010;30:662-673.

Stimulation of dorsal root ganglia for the management of complex regional pain syndrome: a prospective case series.
Van Buyten JP, Smet I, Liem L, Russo M, Huygen F.
Pain Pract. 2015;15:208-216.

Chronic Low Back Pain: Restoration of Dynamic Stability.
Deckers K, De Smedt K, Van Buyten JP, Smet, I., Eldabe, S., Gulve, A., Baranidharan, G., de Andres, J., Gilligan, C., Jaax, K., Heemels, J. P., Crosby, P.
Neuromodulation. 2015;18:478-486

Table of content

Hypotheses 1

Chapter 1: Introduction 2

Which ganglion do we stimulate for chronic pain: current treatment and trends.......................2
- *Abstract*...3
- *Introduction*..4
- *Head and facial pain*...5
- *Spine related pain*...11
- *Conclusions*..19
- *References*...20

Chapter 2: 26

Chronic Stimulation of the Gasserian Ganglion in Patients with Trigeminal Neuropathy: A Case Series 26
- *Abstract*...27
- *Introduction*..28
- *Methods*..29
- *Results*..32
- *Conclusion*..33
- *References*...34

Chapter 3 36

Stimulation of the Gasserian ganglion in the treatment of refractory trigeminal neuropathy 36
- *Abstract*...37
- *Introduction*..38
- *Materials and methods*..39
- *Results*..41
- *Discussion*..47
- *Conclusion*..49
- *References*...51

Chapter 4 54

Electromagnetic Navigation Technology for More Precise Electrode Placement in the Foramen Ovale: A Technical Report 54
- *Abstract*...55
- *Introduction*..56
- *EM Navigation Guided Procedure*..57
- *Discussion*..58

Chapter 5 64

Phenotype of patients responsive to occipital nerve stimulation for refractory head pain............64
- *Abstract*...65
- *Introduction*..66
- *Methods*..66

Results 69
Discussion 77
Conclusion 79
References 80

Chapter 6 84

Stimulation of Dorsal Root Ganglia for the Management of Complex Regional Pain Syndrome: A Prospective Case Series 84

Abstract 85
Introduction 86
Methods 87
Results 88
Conclusions 93
References 94

Chapter 7 100

Chronic Low Back Pain: Restoration of Dynamic Stability 100

Abstract 101
Introduction 102
Materials and methods 104
Results 106
Discussion 111
References 114

Chapter 8 118

General Discussion and Future Perspectives 118

History 119
The dorsal root ganglion an ideal target for neurostimulation 119
Stimulation of the Gasserian ganglion 121
Indirect stimulation of ganglia 121
Future perspectives, need for further research 122
Conclusions 124
References 125

Chapter 9 130

Conclusions/Conclusies 130

Conclusion 131
Conclusie 132

Curriculum vitae 134

List of publications 136

Publications in peer reviewed journals 137
Book chapters 140

Dankwoord / Acknowledgments 142

List of abbreviations

AAC	anterior cingulate cortex
AE	adverse event
AFP	Atypical facial pain
aids	acquired immune deficiency syndrome
ANOVA	Analysis of Variance
AP	antero-posterior
ATP	adenosine-5-triphosphate
BPISF	brief pain inventory short form
BURST DR	burst stimulation according to De Ridder
CGRP	calcitonin gene-related peptide
CLBP	Chronic low back pain
CNS	central nervous system
CRPS	complex regional pain syndrome
CT	Computed tomography
cTN	classic trigeminal neurlagia
CTN	computed tomography
DREZ	dorsal root entry zone
DRG	dorsal root ganglion
EM	electromagnetic
EMG	electromyography
ENT	ear, nose and throat
EQ-5D-3L	Euroquol 5 dimensions'questionnaire
FBSS	failed back surgery syndrome
FDA	food & drug administration
fMRI	functional magnetic resonance imaging
GDP	Gross Domestic Product
GG	Gasserian ganglion
GKR	gamma-knife radiosurgery
HF10	high frequency spinal cord stimulation at 10Kilohertz
HIV	Human immunodeficiency virus
Hz	hertz
IASP	international association for the study of pain
ICHD	international criteria for headache disorders
ICHD	International Classification of Headache Disorders
INDO	Indomethacin
INDO test	Indomethacine test
IPG	internal pulse generator
K	potassium
LM	Lumbar multifidus
	Milli Ampère

mA	
MCI	Motor Control Impairment
mcs	microseconds
MD	Missing Data
mg	milligrams
min	minute
MO	Medication Overuse
MOA	mechanism of action
MOH	medication overuse headache
MR	magnetic resonance
MRI	Magnetic Resonsance Imaging
Na	sodium
NANS	North American Neuromodulation Society
NC	Not Classifiable
NNH	Number needed to harm
NNT	Number needed to treat
NRS	numeric rating scale
NS	neurostimulator
ODI	Oswestry Disability Index
ONS	occipital nerve(field) stimulation
PDPN	painful diabetic polyneuropathy
PET	positron emission tomography
PHN	post herpetic neuralgia
POMS	profile of mood states
PRF	pulsed radiofrequency
QoL	quality of life
RCT	randomized controlled trial
RF	radiofrequency
ROC	region under the curve
SCS	spinal cord stimulation
sec	seconds
SEM	standard error to the mean
SGC	satellite glial cell
SNRI	serotonine noradrenaline reuptake inhibitors
SNT	surgical navigation technology
SS	sandwich synapse
TCA	tricyclic antidepressants
TCC	trigemino cervical complex
	trigeminal deafferentation pain

TDP	
TGS	trigeminal gasserian ganglion stimulation
TN	trigeminal neuralgia
TNF	tumor necrosis factor
TNP	Trigeminal neuropathy
V 1/V2/V3	fifth cranial nerve: first second and third branch
VAS	visual analogue score
μs	micro second

Hypotheses

1) The ganglia are the relay between the peripheral nervous system and the central nervous system and can be stimulated
    a) directly
        The Gasserian ganglion discussed in chapter 2 and 3
        Dorsal root ganglion stimulation discussed in chapter 6
        Pterygopalatine ganglion stimulation discussed in chapter 6
    b) indirectly
        Stimulation of the trigeminal cervical complex discussed in chapter 5
        Medial branch stimulation described in chapter 7

2) The improvement in visualization of the procedure, improves the precision of electrode placement and the safety for the patient and the physician. Discussed in chapter 3 and 8

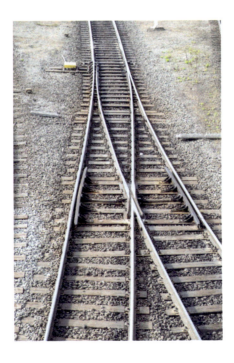

Chapter 1: Introduction
Which ganglion do we stimulate for chronic pain: current treatment and trends

Jean Pierre Van Buyten [1]; Lisa Goudman [2,3]; Maarten Moens [3,4]

1 Multidisciplinary Pain Center, AZ Nikolaas, Sint Niklaas, Belgium
2 Department of Physiotherapy, Human Physiology and Anatomy, Faculty of Physical Education & Physiotherapy, Vrije Universiteit Brussel, Brussels, Belgium & Pain in Motion International Research Group, www.paininmotion.be
3 Dept of Neurosurgery, Universitair Ziekenhuis Brussel, Brussels, Belgium
4 Dept of Radiology, Universitair Ziekenhuis Brussel, Brussels, Belgium

Submitted

Abstract

The treatment of chronic pain syndromes is still challenging. Electrically stimulating the spinal cord has proven to be effective and safe. Considering the different ganglia, stimulation of the Gasserian ganglion reduces trigeminal neuropathic pain, likewise stimulation of the pterygopalatine ganglion and/or stimulation of the occipital nerve is effective in the treatment of cluster headache. Targeting the dorsal root ganglion is simplified by the development of a specific device that has the possibility to specifically stimulate this structure whereby clinical experience suggests better paresthetic coverage than with conventional spinal cord stimulation. In this article, the anatomy of the different structures that are currently stimulated and the evidence of the clinical applications are discussed.

Introduction

Even in the 21st century efficaciously treating chronic pain remains a challenge. The latest developments in the pharmacological management did not result in revolutionary treatment solutions and have a high incidence of side effects that may lead to patient refusal to continue therapy. [1] The studies on pharmacological treatment are predominantly performed in painful diabetic polyneuropathy (PDPN) and post herpetic neuralgia (PHN). Extrapolation of these results to other types of neuropathic pain is difficult and not reliable. But even in PDPN and PHN the Number Needed To Treat is high and Number Needed to Harm is low. [1] One of the first-choice anti-neuropathic drugs, pregabalin, was tested in a randomized placebo controlled study. Placebo had a better effect than pregabalin in acute and chronic sciatica. [2] Pharmacological management, more specific the use of major opioids in non-malignant pain, is expensive for both the patient and the health insurance and loses popularity due to the controversy about efficacy, safety, tolerance, addiction and opioid induced hyperalgesia. Prescription based opioids misuse and abuse resulting in death became an epidemic, with the size of the HIV/aids epidemic in the 80's. Interventional pain management techniques are documented to reduce the need for pharmacological treatment. Moreover, there is a tendency towards a mechanism based treatment approach. [3] Regarding the interventional techniques, neurodestructive interventions are target-specific but have the drawback of being irreversible. Neurostimulation instead is reversible, but paresthesia based tonic spinal cord stimulation can fail to provide satisfactory pain relief because of the incomplete coverage of the painful dermatome, although its efficacy has been proven in the treatment of several pathologies. Direct stimulation of the Gasserian ganglion was already described in 1980 by Meyerson and Hakansson [4] to alleviate trigeminal neuropathy. The stimulation of the occipital nerves was demonstrated to provide pain relief in patients with cluster headache. [5, 6]

A preferred target for the treatment of chronic pain is the DRG due to its accessibility and key function in the transmission and transduction of pain. Dorsal root ganglionectomy was popular during the 1960's and 1970's. Resection of one single mapped DRG was not able to treat the whole painful area because of convergent and divergent pathways. [7] (see figure 1)

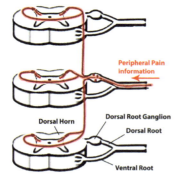

Figure 1: Convergent and divergent pathways through pain in the dorsal root ganglion.
Multisegmental input to similar synaptic location
Segmental input to divergent spinal synaptic location
Red: Peripheral pain information entering via the sensible fibers through the peripheral nerve.

The invasiveness of the treatment and the poor quality of the evidence have made DRG resection less atractive.[8] Radiofrequency and pulsed radiofrequency treatment adjacent to the DRG have been studied at lumbar and cervical level for the management of radicular pain. Radiofrequency treatment adjacent to the lumbar DRG was not better than sham intervention.[9] A prospective trial studying the effect of pulsed radiofrequency adjacent to the lumbar DRG showed clinical success in more than 50% of the patients[10]. Two RCT's demonstrate an effect of radiofrequency treatment adjacent to the cervical DRG. One compared radiofrequency to sham[11] while the second study compared radiofrequency at 60°C with 40°C[12] Pulsed radiofrequency proved to be superior to sham. [13]

New perspectives are opened for the treatment of pain syndromes that are difficult to cover with SCS due to the development of a special device allowing the stimulation of the DRG for the treatment of neuropathic pain syndromes in specific dermatomes. [14-16]

The ganglia, also described as nerve cell clusters, play an important role in the pain transmission and therefore can be suitable targets for neurostimulation whereby **we hypothesize that the ganglia can be stimulated directly as well as indirectly.**

We provide an overview of the most frequently stimulated ganglia, their anatomy and the evidence of ganglion stimulation in chronic pain management.

Head and facial pain

Gasserian or trigeminal ganglion – Direct ganglion stimulation

The Gasserian ganglion has been targeted with neuro-ablative techniques, such as glycerol and radiofrequency, balloon decompression and gamma knife for the treatment of trigeminal neuralgia refractory to conservative treatment. [17] The efficacy of those treatments is variable. The development of chronic trigeminal neuropathic pain is one of the side effects. In these cases, repeat ablative interventions are redundant. The differential diagnosis between trigeminal neuralgia (ICHD 13.1.1) and trigeminal neuropathic pain (ICHD 13.1.2)[18] is extremely important, because the treatment of both diseases is different.

Anatomy of the Gasserian ganglion

The centripetal fibers of the sensory root and the fibers of the motor roots of the 5th cranial nerve enter Meckel's cave or the so-called trigeminal cave (space between two layers of the dura mater (meningeal and periosteal layer)) at the petrous apex through an opening in the dura called the pours trigeminus. [19] The Gasserian ganglion, also called trigeminal ganglion or semilunar ganglion, is situated in the trigeminal cave. [20] This trigeminal cave is covered by the sagittal plate of the cavernous sinus where it merges into the dura of the anterior surface of the petrous part and the tentorium cerebelli.[21] In the cave, surrounding the root bundles of the trigeminal nerve, lays also the arachnoid of the cisterna trigemini.[22] Distal to the ganglion, the trigeminal nerve splits up into his three principal branches; the ophthalmic, maxillary and mandibular nerve.[19] The motor roots are divided into two or three root fibers above the sensory root (superior part) and the inferior motor root, which emerges from the pons in front of the sensory root. The superior and inferior parts join after a course of variable length.[21]

The Gasserian ganglion is a discrete semilunar structure in the inferolateral aspect of Meckel's cave. The convex margin is always oriented inferolateral. The ganglion contains cell bodies of afferent sensory fibers, except fibers that mediate proprioception. [19] The part of the sensory root derived from the ophthalmic nerve usually runs above, the part from the maxillary nerve in the middle and the part from the mandibular nerve in the lower portions.[21] The meningeal investment of the anterior surface of the Gasserian ganglion is very adhesive; on the posterior surface, it is only adherent on the anterior third. [20] The arterial blood supply to the Gasserian ganglion is derived from branches of the intracavernous carotid artery (inferolateral trunk, meningohypophysical trunk or the middle meningeal artery). [22]

The shape of the ganglion varies from thin/regular to thick and nodular. Several studies described the length, thickness and width. Although high variability on the measurement since the morphometry of the skull base and the petrous bone has a high individual variability, the ganglion is 14-22 mm long and approx. 4mm thick.[20, 21, 23]

Indications

Stimulation of the Gasserian ganglion has been reported to control trigeminal neuropathic pain refractory to conservative treatment. The classification based on the patients symptoms and history can help establishing the diagnosis.[24] The indications for stimulation of the Gasserian ganglion are neuropathic pain in the face due to peripheral nerve injury such as trigeminal neuropathic pain (TNP), incidental and non-intentional nerve lesion after ear nose throat, maxilo facial or dental surgery, stroke, and trauma; peripheral nerve injury after ablation (RF, glycerol, gamma knife procedure) or post herpetic neuralgia with a trigeminal distribution

Clinical results

Already in 1978, Steude [25] reported a pain relief lasting from 14 days to 6 weeks in 11 patients after percutaneous electro stimulation of the trigeminal tract.

Meyerson [26] reported on 14 patients who were treated with an implanted electrode into the Gasserian ganglion. The patients were followed for 1- 7 years (mean 4 years). Eleven patients had retained the pain relief and pain disappeared completely in 1 patient without further stimulation. The electrode had to be replaced in several patients because the insulation of the lead wires frequently broke.

In a review of 8 trials on electro stimulation of the Gasserian ganglion in 233 patients with trigeminal neuralgia refractory to conservative treatment, 48% of the patients had at least 50% pain relief. [27]

Mehrkens published the results of more than 300 patients who were followed for a minimum of one year after the implantation of a permanent pulsed generator, once the patients had a positive trial period with an electrode implanted in the foramen ovale. Good to excellent analgesic effect was obtained in 52% of the patients. [28]

In a report of 8 patients suffering trigeminal neuropathy due to trauma, post herpetic neuralgia, surgery or ablative treatments of trigeminal neuralgia, a specially designed electrode to avoid dislocation and dysesthesia was placed under electromagnetic neuronavigation.[29] All patients experienced minimum 30% pain relief during the trial period and requested and received permanent implantation. Subsequently the author report on 22 patients implanted with the custom-made electrode for a trial period lasting at least 4 weeks. In 17 of the 22 patients pain relief justified permanent implantation. Fifteen of the 17 patients had at least 50% pain reduction, the remaining two patients had 44% and 33% pain reduction. The initial VAS score decreased from 9-10 on a 10-point scale to 4/10 at 2 weeks' follow-up and 2/10 at the long-term follow-up (range 4.5 months to 63 months). 88% of the patients could partially or completely stop the use of pain medication. Up to 41% of the patients had dysesthesia and/or physical discomfort, but no major complications requiring device removal were reported. [30]

The use of Electro Magnetic (EM) neuronavigation guidance offers the possibility of a more precise lead placement under "real time" supervision without the need for extra exposure of the patient and the physician to the radiation of continuous fluoroscopy control. [31] Needles suitable for EM navigation, and allowing real time monitoring of the needle placement during percutaneous pain management techniques, have been developed (AZ Nikolaas, Sint- Nikolaas, Belgium in cooperation with the Surgical Navigation Technology, a company based in Denver (Col) USA, presently known as Medtronic-SNT).

The navigation stylet is equipped with two magnetic coils. First a multislice CT-scan is taken of the area between the puncture (entry point) of the skin and the target (the foramen ovale). The best scans where the target is most visible in coronal, axial and sagittal view is downloaded from the hospital network or from an optical disc to the computer of the navigation system. During the procedures, the patient's head is positioned upon a magnet and maintained within a magnetic field. Certain reference points on the three-dimensional reconstruction of the face are ticked into the computer by simple mouse clicks. The same reference points are indicated with a coiled stylet applied to the face and sent to the navigation machine (Stealth station- Medtronic) by touching the face. One reference point (antenna) is fixed to the frontal area of the skull. This point is also entered into the computer, thus situating the position of the patient within the magnetic field, and allowing the patient to move without causing any loss of precision of the representation. The track is dotted out virtually on the computer screen. See Figure 2.

The computer, matching virtual landmarks on the three-dimensional reconstruction of the face with the same landmarks on the patient's face, calculates the operating circle with a precision of approximately 1 mm. The coiled stylet is introduced into the needle and can be navigated towards the foramen ovale following in real time exactly the virtual track. Once the needle passes the foramen a short control of its position is made by a one shot fluoroscopic image not lasting longer than 1 sec. By removing the coiled stylet, we lose contact with the magnetic field and the navigation Station. Because of the real-time visualization of the lead placement the procedure can be performed under local anesthesia or light propofol sedation. [32]

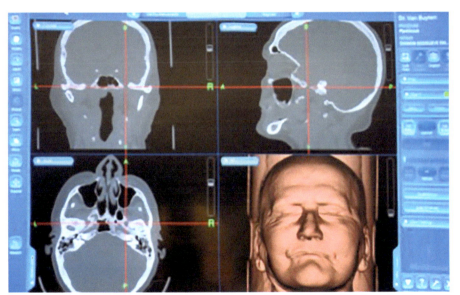

Figure 2: Neuronavigation screen showing the virtual track of the stimulation lead, from the skin to the foramen ovale.

Stimulation of the Gasserian ganglion was shown to be effective in well-selected patients with trigeminal neuropathic pain. The main challenge is the selection of the electrode. A small diameter electrode (0.7 mm) does not induce dysesthesia but the electrode is dislocated in 10 % of the cases. A larger electrode of 0.9 mm did not dislocate but dysesthesia occurred in 18 % of the patients.

The development of a new curved, tined; tripolar electrode design (Medtronic Neurological, Minneapolis, Minnesota, Model 09053) limits retraction and displacement.[29]

The optimization of the technique, with the use of EM neuronavigation guidance reduces the risk of complications. [31]

Summary Gasserian ganglion stimulation

Although the stimulation of the Gasserian ganglion was already described in 1978, the development of an electrode that anchors into the foramen ovale initiated a major improvement of the long-term results, with a serious reduction in the incidence of lead migration. The EM guidance allows a reduction of the intervention time, the patient's discomfort during the treatment, and the radiation exposure for both the patient and the physician.

Studies on larger series should help identify the patients that may have the most benefit. The stimulation of the Gasserian ganglion is a last resort treatment therefore a randomized controlled trial will be extremely hard to perform mainly because of ethical reasons. New stimulation paradigms and wave forms such as burst stimulation, and high frequency stimulation could possibly have an influence on the long-term success and has to be explored.

Trigeminal cervical complex -Indirect Ganglion Stimulation

Occipital nerve stimulation was used for the treatment of occipital neuralgia. [33] The International Headache Society described occipital neuralgia as unilateral or bilateral paroxysmal, shooting or stabbing pain in the posterior part of the scalp, in the distribution of the greater, lesser or third occipital nerves, sometimes accompanied by diminished sensation or dysesthesia in the affected area and commonly associated with tenderness over the involved nerve(s).[34] However, occipital neuralgia is often present together with migraine.[35] Therefore it is possible that patients treated with occipital nerve stimulation were suffering migraine with or without occipital neuralgia. Furthermore, stimulation of the occipital nerve proved to alleviate cluster headache.[5]

The question arises, what do we stimulate when placing the electrode at the major or minor occipital nerve?

Trigeminocervical complex

The trigeminocervical complex (TCC) consists of the rostral 2-3 segments of the cervical spine and the dorsal horns of the medulla.[36] Stimulation of trigeminal nociceptors can clinically be observed by responses in both the trigeminal and cervical regions [37] due to convergence of trigeminal and cervical afferents (input from teeth, muscles of mastication, tempomandibular joint and neck muscles), to the neurons in the TCC. [36, 38] A well-known example is the pain distribution in patients with migraine who experience pain in the front of the head, cutaneously innervated by the trigeminal nerve and pain in the back of the head that is derived from the greater occipital nerve, a branch of the C2 spinal root. [39] Besides the convergence of input, signs of allodynia and hypersensitivity are often reported and can be explained by sensitization of the second order neurons in the TCC which leads to increased excitability over time [39].

The TCC receives his major afferent input from the C2 spinal root that is peripherally represented by the greater occipital nerve. The superficial and deep layers of the dorsal horn of the TCC receive input from A- and C-fiber afferents of the dural and cervical afferents. Recently researchers demonstrated that part of the neurons in the C2 dorsal horn received convergence input from the dura mater and the greater occipital nerve. This means there is a direct anatomical coupling between the cervical and meningeal afferents. Noxious stimulation of the dura mater results in facilitated responses in the greater occipital nerve, which not only confirms the anatomical connection, it also highlights the functional connection. Cervical and dural afferents have an anatomical connection and an important functional connection for mutual changes of excitability. Starting in the TCC, ascending nociceptive pathways project to supraspinal relay sites like the thalamus. The nociceptive input to the second order neurons in the TCC is further modulated by top down inhibitory projections from the brainstem. The rostroventral medulla, nucleus raphe magnus and the periaquaductorial gray are believed to have a key role in this pain modulating circuit. [38, 39] (figure 3)

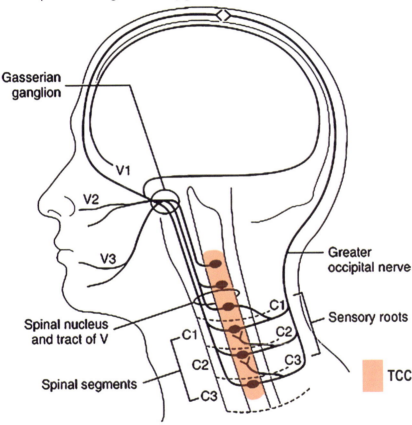

Figure 3: Schematic illustration of the trigeminocervical complex (TCC) marked in red.

Clinical relevance of the TCC

The TCC can be an appropriate target to treat different headache disorders. High cervical epidural stimulation targeting the DREZ of C1 C2 C3 with retrograde placement of the lead resulted in poor success rate. Barolat et al [40] were looking at the effectiveness of SCS in eliciting paresthesias in function of the level of the tip of the lead. The effectiveness of SCS in eliciting paresthesias in the C2 area was less than 20%.

Stimulation of the TCC (=indirect ganglion stimulation) by stimulating the occipital nerve field can be successful in the treatment of different headache disorders. The technique was first introduced by Weiner and Reed[41] who published a series of 8 patients with refractory occipital neuralgia treated successfully with occipital nerve stimulation. Later these patients were reviewed by Peter Goadsby. He diagnosed the patients as migraineurs instead of suffering from occipital neuralgia. (personal communication)

A retrospective study assessed the results of 44 consecutive patients implanted with occipital nerve stimulation for chronic headache with a follow up time of 2.9 years. The authors tried to identify the phenotype of the patients that best responded to ONS. [42] ICHD 13.12, (constant pain caused by compression, irritation or distortion of cranial nerves or upper cervical roots by structural lesions) the so-called cervicogenic headache seems to respond best. Patients suffering from migraine without aura (ICHD 1.1) are also good responders to ONS. Within this group additional medication overuse headache (MOH) (ICHD 8.2) seems to be a predictor for less favorable outcome.

In a PET study Matharu et al [43] showed significant changes in regional cerebral blood flow correlated to pain scores and to stimulation induced paresthesias and documented C1-2-3 paresthesia correlated thalamic activation of pulvinar, cuneous and anterior cingulate cortex (ACC) with ONS, which is consistent with the region activated in episodic migraine.

Treatment of cluster headache

The first line treatment of cluster headache is pharmacological. It is subdivided in acute and prophylactic treatment. Acute treatment can only be used in case of attacks. When the attacks persist, and become chronic, a prophylactic treatment should be considered.

For patients suffering cluster headache refractory to pharmacological treatment interventional treatment modalities may be used. Various destructive procedures of the trigeminal ganglion and/ or the ganglion pterygopalatinum have been used with variable success and risk of devastating side effects and complications. [44]

Neurostimulation techniques are non-destructive and reversible. Deep brain stimulation, occipital nerve stimulation and stimulation of the ganglion pterygopalatinum have been proposed.

Deep brain stimulation is a rather invasive treatment and is out of the scope of this review.

Occipital nerve stimulation

Occipital nerve stimulation was first reported for the treatment of occipital neuralgia. [41] The stimulation targets are the distal branches of the C2-C3 roots corresponding with the greater and lesser occipital nerves. In this way, the stimulation of the TCC is indirect ganglion stimulation.

Several case series and observational studies on the use of occipital nerve stimulation for the treatment of cluster headache have been reported. [5, 45-54]

The first patients of a series of 14 received a unilateral implant with good effect, but side shift in pain. The following patients were bilaterally implanted. Ten out of 14 patients showed improvement but none had complete pain relief. [45, 46] A second case series including 15 patients who received unilateral implanted occipital nerve stimulation showed that 80% of the patients had a 90% improvement and 60% was pain free for prolonged periods. [5, 6]

In a case series of 15 headache patients, 3 had cluster headache refractory to drug treatment. Two received unilateral and one bilateral stimulation of the occipital nerve. After 20 months 2 of the 3 patients improved. [48, 49]

In a series of 7 patients 6 experienced a positive effect, with a reduction of the intensity and frequency of the attacks to about 50% of baseline. All responders could reduce the attack medication by 77%. [51]

Comparable success rates were reported by de Quintana-Schmidt[52], who reported 4 cases, and Strand [54], who implanted a rechargeable micro stimulator in 3 patients.

Wolter [55] implanted epidural electrodes high in the cervical region. After a mean follow up of 23 months all patients experienced reduction in frequency, duration and intensity of the attacks. The positive effect was observed immediately after the electrode implantation.

With occipital nerve stimulation, paresthesia is felt along the greater occipital nerve region, which was well tolerated by the patients who had a positive effect, but is reported to be unbearable by one patient who had no effect.

Summary TCC

The TCC may be a potential target for the treatment of different types of headache. The available evidence is rather weak, because of the different types of headache, and the low number of patients included. It is noticed that the effect of the stimulation may only be felt after several weeks.

There is need for more studies that identify the patients who would benefit most from this treatment. Therefore, work needs to be done on the patient inclusion criteria.

The role of neurostimulation in the management of headache is supported by the statement in a consensus article from the European Headache Federation, [56] that neurostimulation should be considered once all alternative drug and behavioral therapies failed and MOH is excluded.

It is recommended to start with the least invasive stimulation method and move on to more invasive approaches when the headache proves to be refractory.

Spine related pain

The dorsal root ganglion – direct ganglion stimulation

The dorsal root ganglion (DRG) has been described as gate keeper, a railway marshaling station, a highway intersection... All these terms indicate the key role of the DRG in relaying sensory information from the periphery to the central nervous system (CNS). With tonic SCS paresthesias covering the painful area are researched. Unfortunately, this is not always possible.

Anatomy of the DRG

The right and left paired "mixed" spinal nerves carry autonomic, motor and sensory information between the periphery and the spinal cord. These spinal nerves are composed of afferent sensory dorsal axons (dorsal root) and motor ventral efferent axons (ventral root). They emerge from the intervertebral neural foramina between adjacent vertebral segments.[57,58] The dorsal sensory roots exit the neural foramina to form the DRG.

The DRG is located bilaterally on the distal end of the dorsal root in the antero-lateral epidural space. In men, there are 8-paired cervical, 12 paired thoracic, 5 paired lumbar and 4-paired sacral DRGs. The morphology of the DRG is longer and wider as it is more caudally located. (Figure 4)

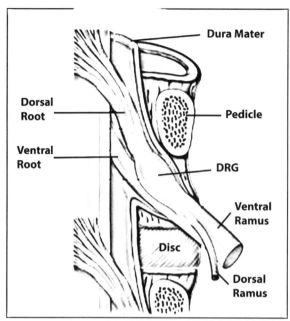

Figure 4: Schematic illustration of the dorsal root ganglion.
DRG: Dorsal Root Ganglion

At the cervical level the DRG is located in the superolateral part of the foramen, [59] in the nerve root groove, posteriorly and medially to the vertebral artery [60] and between the vertebral artery and a concavity in the superior articular process [61]. Mostly, the vertebral artery enters the foramen transversarius at the level of C6 to serve as the parent vessel for several segmental medullary vessels. This close relationship of the segmental medullary vessels with the DRG is important to understand the possible impact on targeting the DRG for therapeutic purposes.[62] The intervertebral foramen is anteriorly defined by the uncinate process, posteriorly by the superior facet joint and the pedicles form the superior and inferior bounders. [59, 61] In healthy individuals the DRGs from L1 to L3 are mostly foraminal, L4 lays foraminal. At L5 the DRG lays foraminal or, in a minority of the cases, intraspinal.[63]

The DRG consists of a collection of bipolar cell bodies of primary sensory neurons surrounded by glial cells and the axons of the DRG sensory cells that form the primary afferent sensory nerve. The DRG neurons are pseudo unipolar neurons composed of two branches, a distal and a proximal process, connected by an outgrowth cell body.

The DRG contains the largest proportion of sensory nerves of the body. These cells are responsible for the transduction of visceral and somatic sensory information from the periphery and transmitting this information to the CNS. The cell bodies actively participate in the signaling process by sensing certain molecules and manufacturing other molecules that modulate the sensory transduction process [64]. They are surrounded by layers of satellite glial cells (SGCs).

The DRG is not protected by a blood nerve barrier, allowing small and large molecules and even macrophages to cross the SGC wrap of the DRG neuron.[65]

Satellite glial cells form a functional unit of the sensory neuron within the DRG, the glial cells tell the nervous system what to do.[66] Stimulation of the DRG neuron triggers a delayed and long-lasting response by a pathway between glia, called the "sandwich synapse" (SS).[67] The receptors on the SGCs such as chemokines, cytokines, adenosine-5'-triphosphate (ATP), bradykinins participate in the transmission process of within the DRG. Glial cells change in morphology and biochemical function after a peripheral afferent fiber injury and participate actively in the central and peripheral nervous system processes.

The role of the DRG in impulse propagation

Primary sensory neurons start at the peripheral receptive field of the neuron, and have their cell body in the DRG. A stimulus in the periphery alters the firing of the neuron and propagates into the CNS, beginning in the dorsal horn of the spinal cord and ending in the relevant portions of the thalamus and brain.[68] The pseudo uni-polar neurons of the DRG lie within the DRG and have axons that split peripherally and centrally away from the soma. At the branch point, the so-called T-junction the DRG can act as an impediment to electrical impulse from the nociceptor to the dorsal root entry zone specifically, it can gate the propagation of the electrical pulse by acting as a low pass filter to electrical information from the periphery.[69] (Figure 5)

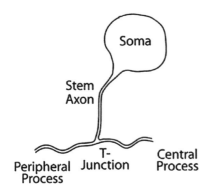

Figure 5: Impulse propagation and role of the T-junction.

Thermo-mechanical reception occurs in small unmyelinated, nociceptive C-fiber cells in the DRG. These cells contain substance-P or calcitonin gene-related peptide (CGRP), which they use as neuromodulators and neurotransmitters. The terminals of the larger, myelinated A-fiber neurons are low-threshold mechanoreceptors. [70]

When primary sensory neurons are injured, Schwann cells and SGCs in the DRG release pro-inflammatory mediators such as eicosanoids, bradykinins, serotonin, neurotrophins, cytokines such interleukins, TNF-α, interferons, growth factors, chemokines, ATP and reactive oxygen species. [70]

Ion channels and receptors that are located in the primary sensory neurons have three functions: transduction, transmission, and modulation of sensory information. Transduction of noxious information to electrical signals at the peripheral terminals of the DRG includes, transient receptor potential channels, Na+ channels, acid-sensing ion channels, and ATP-sensitive receptors. [71] Propagation of action potentials involves Na+ and K+ channels, while voltage-gated Ca++ channels and glutamate receptors perform the modulation of synaptic transmission. The latter are expressed on presynaptic membranes at the terminal of the primary afferents of the dorsal horn.

Somatotopy of the DRG

The cell bodies within the DRG are somatotopically organized. The topographical distribution of sciatic and femoral nerve sensory neuronal somata in the L4 dorsal root ganglion of the adult rat was mapped after retrograde tracing. (Figure 6) The tracers were applied to the proximal transected end of either nerve alone, or from both nerves in the same animal using separate tracers. Three-dimensional reconstructions of the distribution of labeled neurons were made from serial sections of the L4 dorsal root ganglion, which is the only ganglion that these two nerves share. The results showed that with little overlap, femoral nerve neurons distribute dorsally and rostrally whereas sciatic nerve neurons distribute medially and ventrally. This finding indicates the existence of a somatotopical organization for the representation of different peripheral nerves in dorsal root ganglia of adult animals.[72] Theoretically this makes it possible to specify the target.

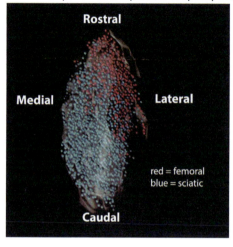

Figure 6: Somatotopic arrangement in the L4 DRG
blue: sciatic nerve ; red: femoral nerve.

Potential indications for DRG stimulation

The target specific stimulation allows coverage of dermatomes that are difficult to access by stimulation of the dorsal horns of the spinal cord, such as the extremities.

DRG stimulation has an impact on the autonomic function. Stimulation of the afferent neurons can produce a reflex arc involving interneurons that project to the intermediolateral cell column housing sympathetic pre-motor neurons. Both spinal and supraspinal regions modulate this reflex which can induce potent and regional sympatholytic effects. Reduction of sympathetic outflow can result in peripheral vasodilation and so impact vasculature and sympathetically associated pain mechanism such as in CRPS.

We also know that the DRG's are connected to the sympathetic chain, so direct stimulation of the DRG must physically have an impact on the sympathetic nervous system (Figure 7)

Therefore, DRG stimulation may be envisioned in the management of chronic low back and limb pain, essentially in the L5S1 dermatomes, potentially after back surgery treatment or CRPS, neuropathic pain due to nerve injury such as post herpetic neuralgia; post mastectomy pain, inguinal neuralgia, thoracotomy, and neuropathic pain in the extremities, arm, hand, leg and foot (ex neuropathic pain due to post ganglionic brachial plexus elongation). Due to convergent and divergent pathways, multi-segmental stimulation of non-adjacent levels is often employed to obtain coverage over a wide range of dermatomes.

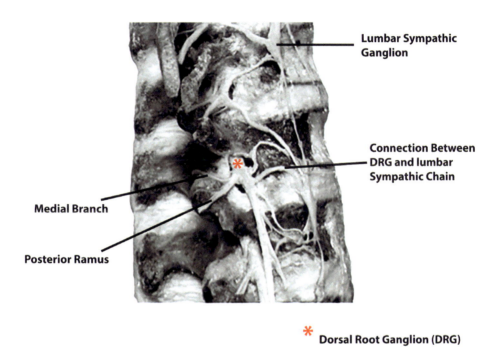

Figure 7: Anatomic preparation of the dorsal root ganglion.

Clinical results

A pilot study on 10 patients with chronic pain of the back and the limbs showed that DRG stimulation reduced the pain in almost 90% of the patients with at least 30%. More than 70% of the patients could reduce the need for analgesic medication. The authors observed pain relief in specific anatomical regions such as the leg, back, and foot, that are difficult to reach with SCS.[16]

In a multicenter, prospective study 51 patients with chronic intractable pain received a trial implantation. At the end of the trial period 39 patients reported more than 50% pain relief. Seven patients did not proceed to implanted stimulation; 2 did not give a reason for refusal, in 1 patient pain did not recur since trial implantation, another patient had 100 % pain relief in one foot but none in the other, 3 patients were withdrawn for other medical reasons. Thirty-two patients received an implanted stimulator. All had chronic neuropathic pain of varying etiology, most frequent diagnoses were CRPS and FBSS and diverse neuropathic pain conditions. [73] One week after the permanent implantation the patients' average pain was reduced from 77. 6 mm (baseline) to 34.9 mm on a 100 mm VAS scale. The average pain at 4 weeks was 36.6 mm. At 4-week assessment the stimulation was suspended to verify intra-subject effectiveness. After one week without stimulation the patients reported that the overall pain returned to near-baseline levels. The stimulation was restored and at 2 months post-implant the mean pain level was 39.5 and at 3 months the average pain was 38.4. At 6 months' pain was reported to be 33.5. [73]

The 12-month follow-up of these patients was published in 2015. [74] Pain was reduced by 56% and 60% of the patients reported improvement greater than 50% in their pain. Quality of life and mood were also improved and patients reported a high degree of satisfaction. The good pain-paresthesia overlapping at the time of implantation remained stable over the 12-month follow-up study.

A case report on the DRG stimulation for the management of CRPS type I of the knee illustrates the possibility to obtain full coverage with DRG stimulation. [75] Implantation of DRG stimulation lead at L3 did not result in entire coverage of the painful area. Implantation of a lead at L4 improved coverage, though this was not complete; following an additional lead implantation at L2 the coverage was almost complete. After 8 days of stimulation the patient reported a substantial pain relief but a spot at the lateral knee was not covered. The patient was satisfied with the degree of pain reduction from NRS 6-9 at baseline to NRS 1; therefore, the permanent pulse generator was implanted. At one-month post implantation the patient reported entire coverage of the painful area and a NRS score of 1-2. Switching off the stimulator made the pain return within minutes, but switching it back on also produced pain relieving effects within one minute.

In a multicenter prospective trial, patients with CRPS refractory to conservative treatment received a quadripolar percutaneous lead implantation near the DRG relevant to their pain distribution.[76] Patients who had minimum 50 % pain relief during trial stimulation received a permanent implant for 4 weeks. At that point, the stimulator was switched off for one week. During the stimulation period the patients experienced on average 82% pain reduction. When the stimulator was turned off the average pain rebounded to approximately base line value. At 12 months' follow-up, more than 80% of the patients had a pain relief of 50% or higher. Additionally, to the pain reduction, patients reported decreased mood disturbance such as tension, depression, and anger. Patients reported a complete paresthesia coverage of the painful area, which was not different whether the patient was in upright or supine position. Neurovascular changes and improvement in mobility were also reported.

Chronic groin pain may seriously encompass the patient's quality of life and proves often to be refractory to pharmacological, surgical neurectomy and interventional pain treatment. Peripheral nerve stimulation and SCS have been used with varying success. Treatment failure was mainly due to the difficulty in finding the lead placement to cover the painful area. In the studies on neuropathic pain management with DRG stimulation [74] some patients with groin pain were included. Finding the exact target level may also be challenging because the sensory input of the groin is covered by nerve fibers derived from L3 up to T11. In a case study a practical workup using retrograde transforaminal paresthesia mapping was performed prior to DRG lead placement. [77]

Under fluoroscopic control, a 22-gauge SMK needle was placed via the retrograde transforaminal approach close to the DRG. After insertion of a thermocouple, paresthesia was elicited by electro-stimulation at 50 Hz and 1 msec pulse width. Patients were asked to describe the location and percentage of the covered painful area. In the operating room the DRG lead was placed at the levels determined by the preoperative paresthesia mapping. DRG stimulation of the pre-operative paresthesia mapping was performed in 3 patients, whereby they all reported more than 90% pain relief.

A retrospective chart review was performed at 11 sites in Europe of patients treated with DRG stimulation for chronic refractory neuropathic pain of the groin. Twenty-nine patients, mostly with post-surgical pain (12 post herniorrhaphy) were included. The patients received up to 3 leads to cover the painful area. Twenty-five patients had a positive trial and received a permanent implant. The mean follow-up period was 27.8 weeks (range 0-68 weeks). At follow-up 80% of the patients had more than 50% pain reduction and 50% had an improvement rate of more than 80%.

The paresthesia coverage in this difficult patient group proved to be specific and avoiding extraneous coverage. Changes in paresthesia were limited, despite changes in position and changes over time. [78]

There are about 50 treatment possibilities described for phantom pain suggesting the refractory nature of the condition. The poor somatotopic specificity is suggested to be the reason for the variable success rates obtained with SCS.

DRG stimulation leads were implanted in 8 patients with phantom limb pain after a positive trial period. Baseline VAS pain score was 85. 5 mm. At a mean follow-up period of 14. 4 months' pain was rated to be 43.5 mm. Patients perception of quality of life and functional capacity improved and some patients could reduce or stop pain medication. Patients reported precise concordance of paresthesia with the painful regions, including their phantom limb. [79]

DRG stimulation could possibly also be effective in the treatment of low back pain. It has been reported that one of the main pathways of pain originating from the disc, facet joints and sacroiliac joints is the sympathetic trunk through the L2 spinal nerve root. Back pain could be referred pain in the L2 dermatome. (Figure 8) There are some cases of low back pain reporting the beneficial effect of L2 DRG stimulation. More recently a randomized controlled trial comparing DRG stimulation to traditional SCS in patients with foot pain due to CRPS I, and CRPS II showed superiority in all aspects for DRG stimulation. On 152 patients, average pain reduction at 12 months of DRG therapy was 81,4%. 74,2% of the DRG stimulated patients met the primary endpoint (>50% pain relief) at 12 months.[80]

Summary DRG stimulation

In summary, besides the beneficial effects of DRG stimulation, many patients report that subthreshold stimulation is as effective as paresthesia based stimulation. Moreover, there is no positional effect on paresthesias when stimulating the DRG, which makes this neurostimulation technique very convenient for patients. [81]

Direct stimulation on the DRG needs very few energy, resulting in a very long battery lifetime. This makes the therapy less expensive than spinal cord stimulation.

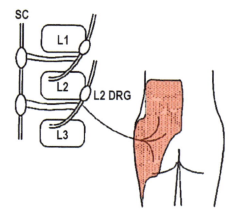

Figure 8: Pathway of pain originating from the disc, facet joints and sacroiliac joints; through sympathetic afferents of the L2 spinal nerve root.
DRG: Dorsal Root Ganglion

Medial branch stimulation – indirect stimulation

Anatomy of the lumbar multifidus muscles

The lumbar multifidus (LM) has a major role in the local stability of the lumbar spine [82, 83] Functionally, the LM is divided into deep, intermediate and superficial fibers, with deep fibers spanning two vertebral segments and functioning tonically, and intermediate and superficial fibers spanning three to five levels and functioning phasically[84, 85] The deep fibers of the LM are anatomically and biomechanically well suited both to provide feedback regarding the position of the spine (proprioception) and, in turn, provide stabilization of the spine. Pain in a joint has been shown to reduce neural drive to the muscles that stabilize the joint. This is known as reflex inhibition. The phenomenon of reflex inhibition is due to an inhibitory process involving afferent discharge from the mechanoreceptors or nociceptors in the joint structures. [86] Local injury to spinal structures leads to reduction in neural drive in the LM, as known by a reduced electric activity. [87, 88] MRI studies suggest that patients suffering from chronic low back pain are more likely to have atrophy of the LM.

The effect of medial branch stimulation

Electronic stimulation of the medial branch of the dorsal ramus with an implanted device, causes the LM to contract episodically, thereby overriding the reflex inhibition

Clinical results

A feasibility study [89] included 26 patients with chronic low back pain refractory to physical therapy and medication. Patients received an implantable pulse generator and leads were positioned adjacent to the medial branch of the dorsal ramus as it crosses the L3 transverse process. Stimulation resulted in contraction of the LM. Patients self-administered stimulation twice daily for 20 min. Three months after treatment start 74% of the patients showed a pain reduction and 63% had an improved disability. Quality of life improved in 84% if the patients. The most frequently encountered problem was lead migration. Interestingly, we observed pain reduction after a few days of stimulation, while the muscle strength could not be restored. We assume that the stimulation of the medial branch is an indirect stimulation of the dorsal root ganglion, which is known to reduce neuropathic pain.

Summary medial branch stimulation

The medial branch of the dorsal ramus is the treatment target for RF heat lesioning in patients with pain originating from the lumbar facet joints. The stimulation applied in the feasibility study has no neurolytic effect, therefore another mechanism of action must interfere with the pain sensation, certainly in the early phase. The muscle stimulation overrides the reflex inhibition and stimulates strength. More research should be performed to confirm these findings.

Conclusions

The development of a device that allows targeting a specific DRG has helped in treating patients with chronic pain syndromes that follow a well-defined dermatome. Likewise, the stimulation of the Gasserian ganglion has offered pain relief and improvement of the quality of life of patients suffering trigeminal neuropathy.

Headache and specifically chronic headache such as cluster headache, migraine, cervicogenic headache and the variety of persistent idiopathic headache syndromes form a challenge for the treating physician. Stimulation of the occipital nerve was documented to be successful in certain types of patients. Although this treatment can be considered as peripheral nerve stimulation, anatomical studies reveal that the ganglia are indirectly stimulated.

It becomes obvious that the ganglia play an important role in the pain transmission, but also the coupling between the TCC and the cervical and meningeal afferents.

These observations give rise to paradigms of ganglionic neurostimulation for the treatment of chronic pain syndromes.

References

1 Finnerup NB, Attal N, Haroutounian S, et al. Pharmacotherapy for neuropathic pain in adults: a systematic review and meta-analysis. *Lancet Neurol*. 2015;14:162-173.
2 Mathieson S, Maher CG, McLachlan AJ, et al. Trial of Pregabalin for Acute and Chronic Sciatica. *New England Journal of Medicine*. 2017;376:1111-1120.
3 Woolf CJ, Bennett GJ, Doherty M, et al. Towards a mechanism-based classification of pain? *Pain*. 1998;77:227-229.
4 Meyerson BA, Hakansson S. Alleviation of atypical trigeminal pain by stimulation of the Gasserian ganglion via an implanted electrode. *Acta Neurochir Suppl (Wien)*. 1980;30:303-309.
5 Magis D, Gerardy PY, Remacle JM, Schoenen J. Sustained effectiveness of occipital nerve stimulation in drug-resistant chronic cluster headache. *Headache*. 2011;51:1191-1201.
6 Magis D, Schoenen J. Occipital nerve stimulation for intractable chronic cluster headache: new hope for a dreadful disease? *Acta neurologica Belgica*. 2011;111:18-21.
7 Osgood CP, Dujovny M, Faille R, Abassy M. Microsurgical lumbosacral ganglionectomy, anatomic rationale, and surgical results. *Acta Neurochir (Wien)*. 1976;35:197-204.
8 Deer T, Levy RM, Kramer JM. Interventional perspectives on the dorsal root ganglion as a target for the treatment of chronic pain: a review. *Minimally Invasive Surgery for Pain*. 2014;2.
9 Geurts JW, van Wijk RM, Wynne HJ, et al. Radiofrequency lesioning of dorsal root ganglia for chronic lumbosacral radicular pain: a randomised, double-blind, controlled trial. *Lancet*. 2003;361:21-26.
10 Van Boxem K, de Meij N, Kessels A, Van Kleef M, Van Zundert J. Pulsed radiofrequency for chronic intractable lumbosacral radicular pain: a six-month cohort study. *Pain Med*. 2015;16:1155-1162.
11 van Kleef M, Liem L, Lousberg R, Barendse G, Kessels F, Sluijter M. Radiofrequency lesion adjacent to the dorsal root ganglion for cervicobrachial pain: a prospective double blind randomized study. *Neurosurgery*. 1996;38:1127-1131; discussion 1131-1122.
12 Slappendel R, Crul BJ, Braak GJ, et al. The efficacy of radiofrequency lesioning of the cervical spinal dorsal root ganglion in a double blinded randomized study: no difference between 40 degrees C and 67 degrees C treatments. *Pain*. 1997;73:159-163.
13 Van Zundert J, Huntoon M, Patijn J, Lataster A, Mekhail N, van Kleef M. 4. Cervical radicular pain. *Pain Pract*. 2009;10:1-17.
14 Koopmeiners AS, Mueller S, Kramer J, Hogan QH. Effect of electrical field stimulation on dorsal root ganglion neuronal function. *Neuromodulation*. 2013;16:304-311; discussion 310-301.
15 Lynch PJ, McJunkin T, Eross E, Gooch S, Maloney J. Case report: successful epiradicular peripheral nerve stimulation of the C2 dorsal root ganglion for postherpetic neuralgia. *Neuromodulation*. 2011;14:58-61; discussion 61.
16 Deer TR, Grigsby E, Weiner RL, Wilcosky B, Kramer JM. A prospective study of dorsal root ganglion stimulation for the relief of chronic pain. *Neuromodulation*. 2013;16:67-71; discussion 71-62.
17 Zakrzewska JM, Akram H. Neurosurgical interventions for the treatment of classical trigeminal neuralgia. *Cochrane Database Syst Rev*. 2011;9:CD007312.

18 Society IH: https://www.ichd-3.org/ 2016. Accessed:
19 Hutchins LG, Harnsberger HR, Hardin CW, Dillon WP, Smoker WR, Osborn AG. The radiologic assessment of trigeminal neuropathy. *AJR Am J Roentgenol*. 1989;153:1275-1282.
20 Arslan M, Deda H, Avci E, et al. Anatomy of Meckel's cave and the trigeminal ganglion: anatomical landmarks for a safer approach to them. *Turkish neurosurgery*. 2012;22:317-323.
21 Lang J. *Clinical Anatomy of the Head*: Springer-Verlag Berlin Heidelberg New York 1983.
22 Downs DM, Damiano TR, Rubinstein D. Gasserian ganglion: appearance on contrast-enhanced MR. *AJNR Am J Neuroradiol*. 1996;17:237-241.
23 Henderson WR. The anatomy of the gasserian ganglion and the distribution of pain in relation to injections and operations for trigeminal neuralgia. *Ann R Coll Surg Engl*. 1965;37:346-373.
24 Burchiel KJ. A new classification for facial pain. *Neurosurgery*. 2003;53:1164-1166; discussion 1166-1167.
25 Steude U. Percutaneous electro stimulation of the trigeminal nerve in patients with atypical trigeminal neuralgia. *Neurochirurgia*. 1978;21:66-69.

26	Meyerson BA, Hakanson S. Suppression of pain in trigeminal neuropathy by electric stimulation of the gasserian ganglion. *Neurosurgery*. 1986;18:59-66.
27	Holsheimer J. Electrical stimulation of the trigeminal tract in chronic, intractable facial neuralgia. *Arch Physiol Biochem*. 2001;109:304-308.
28	Mehrkens JH, Steude U. Chronic electrostimulation of the trigeminal ganglion in trigeminal neuropathy: current state and future prospects. *Acta Neurochir Suppl*. 2007;97:91-97.
29	Van Buyten JP, Hens C. Chronic stimulation of the Gasserian ganglion in patients with trigeminal neuropathy: A case series. *J of Neurosurgical review*. 2011;1:73-77.
30	Kustermans L, Van Buyten JP, Smet I, Coucke W, Politis C. Stimulation of the Gasserian ganglion in the treatment of refractory trigeminal neuropathy. *J Craniomaxillofac Surg*. 2016.
31	Van Buyten JP, Linderoth B. Invasive neurostimulation in facial pain and headache syndromes. *European Journal of Pain Supplements*. 2011;5:409-421.
32	Van Buyten J, Smet I, Van de Kelft E. Electromagnetic Navigation Technology for More Precise Electrode Placement in the Foramen Ovale: A Technical Report *Neuromodulation*. 2009;12:244-249.
33	Goadsby PJ, Bartsch T, Dodick DW. Occipital nerve stimulation for headache: mechanisms and efficacy. *Headache*. 2008;48:313-318.
34	Headache Classification Committee of the International Headache S. The International Classification of Headache Disorders, 3rd edition (beta version). *Cephalalgia*. 2013;33:629-808.
35	Sahai-Srivastava S, Zheng L. Occipital neuralgia with and without migraine: difference in pain characteristics and risk factors. *Headache*. 2011;51:124-128.
36	Panneton WM, Gan Q, Livergood RS. A trigeminoreticular pathway: implications in pain. *PLoS One*. 2011;6:e24499.
37	Park J, Trinh VN, Sears-Kraxberger I, Li KW, Steward O, Luo ZD. Synaptic ultrastructure changes in trigeminocervical complex posttrigeminal nerve injury. *The Journal of comparative neurology*. 2016;524:309-322.
38	Bartsch T, Goadsby PJ. The trigeminocervical complex and migraine: current concepts and synthesis. *Curr Pain Headache Rep*. 2003;7:371-376.
39	Bartsch T. Migraine and the neck: new insights from basic data. *Curr Pain Headache Rep*. 2005;9:191-196.

40	Barolat G, Massaro F, He J, Zeme S, Ketcik B. Mapping of sensory responses to epidural stimulation of the intraspinal neural structures in man. *J Neurosurg*. 1993;78:233-239.
41	Weiner RL, Reed KL. Peripheral neurostimulation for control of intractable occipital neuralgia. *Neuromodulation*. 1999;2:217-221.
42	Paemeleire K, Van Buyten JP, Van Buynder M, et al. Phenotype of patients responsive to occipital nerve stimulation for refractory head pain. *Cephalalgia*. 2010;30:662-673.
43	Matharu MS, Bartsch T, Ward N, Frackowiak RS, Weiner R, Goadsby PJ. Central neuromodulation in chronic migraine patients with suboccipital stimulators: a PET study. *Brain*. 2004;127:220-230.
44	Pedersen JL, Barloese M, Jensen RH. Neurostimulation in cluster headache: a review of current progress. *Cephalalgia*. 2013;33:1179-1193.
45	Burns B, Watkins L, Goadsby PJ. Treatment of medically intractable cluster headache by occipital nerve stimulation: long-term follow-up of eight patients. *Lancet*. 2007;369:1099-1106.
46	Burns B, Watkins L, Goadsby PJ. Treatment of intractable chronic cluster headache by occipital nerve stimulation in 14 patients. *Neurology*. 2009;72:341-345.
47	Magis D, Allena M, Bolla M, De Pasqua V, Remacle JM, Schoenen J. Occipital nerve stimulation for drug-resistant chronic cluster headache: a prospective pilot study. *Lancet Neurol*. 2007;6:314-321.
48	Schwedt TJ, Dodick DW, Hentz J, Trentman TL, Zimmerman RS. Occipital nerve stimulation for chronic headache--long-term safety and efficacy. *Cephalalgia*. 2007;27:153-157.
49	Schwedt TJ, Dodick DW, Trentman TL, Zimmerman RS. Occipital nerve stimulation for chronic cluster headache and hemicrania continua: pain relief and persistence of autonomic features. *Cephalalgia*. 2006;26:1025-1027.
50	Schwedt TJ, Dodick DW, Trentman TL, Zimmerman RS. Response to occipital nerve block is not useful in predicting efficacy of occipital nerve stimulation. *Cephalalgia*. 2007;27:271-274.
51	Muller OM GC, Katsarava Z, Sure U, Diener HC, Gasser T. Bilateral occipital nerve stimulation for the treatment of chronic cluster headache: case series and initiation of a prospective study. *Forthschr Neurol Psychiatr*. 2010;78:709-714.
52	de Quintana-Schmidt C, Casajuana-Garreta E, Molet-Teixido J, et al. [Stimulation of the occipital nerve in the treatment of drug-resistant cluster headache]. *Rev Neurol*. 2010;51:19-26.
53	Fontaine D, Christophe Sol J, Raoul S, et al. Treatment of refractory chronic cluster headache by chronic occipital nerve stimulation. *Cephalalgia*. 2011;31:1101-1105.

54 Strand NH, Trentman TL, Vargas BB, Dodick DW. Occipital nerve stimulation with the Bion(R) microstimulator for the treatment of medically refractory chronic cluster headache. *Pain Physician*. 2011;14:435-440.
55 Wolter T, Kiemen A, Kaube H. High cervical spinal cord stimulation for chronic cluster headache. *Cephalalgia*. 2011;31:1170-1180.
56 Martelletti P, Jensen RH, Antal A, et al. Neuromodulation of chronic headaches: position statement from the European Headache Federation. *J Headache Pain*. 2013;14:86.
57 Hasegawa T, Mikawa Y, Watanabe R, An HS. Morphometric analysis of the lumbosacral nerve roots and dorsal root ganglia by magnetic resonance imaging. *Spine*. 1996;21:1005-1009.
58 Sheng SR, Wang XY, Xu HZ, Zhu GQ, Zhou YF. Anatomy of large animal spines and its comparison to the human spine: a systematic review. *Eur Spine J*. 2010;19:46-56.

59 Ahmed SH, El-Shaarawy EA, Ishaq MF, Moniem MH. Morphological and radiometrical study of the human intervertebral foramina of the cervical spine. *Folia morphologica*. 2014;73:7-18.
60 Tanaka N, Fujimoto Y, An HS, Ikuta Y, Yasuda M. The anatomic relation among the nerve roots, intervertebral foramina, and intervertebral discs of the cervical spine. *Spine*. 2000;25:286-291.
61 Sioutas G, Kapetanakis S. Clinical anatomy and clinical significance of the cervical intervertebral foramen: a review. *Folia morphologica*. 2015.
62 Huntoon MA. Anatomy of the cervical intervertebral foramina: vulnerable arteries and ischemic neurologic injuries after transforaminal epidural injections. *Pain*. 2005;117:104-111.
63 Shen J, Wang HY, Chen JY, Liang BL. Morphologic analysis of normal human lumbar dorsal root ganglion by 3D MR imaging. *AJNR Am J Neuroradiol*. 2006;27:2098-2103.
64 Devor M. Unexplained peculiarities of the dorsal root ganglion. *Pain*. 1999;Suppl 6:S27-35.
65 Hu P, McLachlan EM. Macrophage and lymphocyte invasion of dorsal root ganglia after peripheral nerve lesions in the rat. *Neuroscience*. 2002;112:23-38.
66 Nedergaard M, Ransom B, Goldman SA. New roles for astrocytes: redefining the functional architecture of the brain. *Trends Neurosci*. 2003;26:523-530.
67 Rozanski GM, Li Q, Stanley EF. Transglial transmission at the dorsal root ganglion sandwich synapse: glial cell to postsynaptic neuron communication. *The European journal of neuroscience*. 2013;37:1221-1228.
68 Aldskogius H, Elfvin LG, Forsman CA. Primary sensory afferents in the inferior mesenteric ganglion and related nerves of the guinea pig. An experimental study with anterogradely transported wheat germ agglutinin-horseradish peroxidase conjugate. *J Auton Nerv Syst*. 1986;15:179-190.
69 Gemes G, Koopmeiners A, Rigaud M, et al. Failure of action potential propagation in sensory neurons: mechanisms and loss of afferent filtering in C-type units after painful nerve injury. *J Physiol*. 2013;591:1111-1131.
70 Krames ES. The role of the dorsal root ganglion in the development of neuropathic pain. . *Pain Med*. 2014;15:1669-1685.
71 Reichling DB, Levine JD. Critical role of nociceptor plasticity in chronic pain. *Trends Neurosci*. 2009;32:611-618.
72 Puigdellivol-Sanchez A, Prats-Galino A, Ruano-Gil D, Molander C. Sciatic and femoral nerve sensory neurones occupy different regions of the L4 dorsal root ganglion in the adult rat. *Neurosci Lett*. 1998;251:169-172.
73 Liem L, Russo M, Huygen FJ, et al. A multicenter, prospective trial to assess the safety and performance of the spinal modulation dorsal root ganglion neurostimulator system in the treatment of chronic pain. *Neuromodulation*. 2013;16:471-482; discussion 482.
74 Liem L, Russo M, Huygen FJ, et al. One-year outcomes of spinal cord stimulation of the dorsal root ganglion in the treatment of chronic neuropathic pain. *Neuromodulation*. 2015;18:41-48; discussion 48-49.
75 van Bussel CM, Stronks DL, Huygen FJ. Successful treatment of intractable complex regional pain syndrome type I of the knee with dorsal root ganglion stimulation: a case report. *Neuromodulation*. 2015;18:58-60; discussion 60-51.
76 Van Buyten JP, Smet I, Liem L, Russo M, Huygen F. Stimulation of dorsal root ganglia for the management of complex regional pain syndrome: a prospective case series. *Pain Pract*. 2015;15:208-216.

77 Zuidema X, Breel J, Wille F. Paresthesia mapping: a practical workup for successful implantation of the dorsal root ganglion stimulator in refractory groin pain. *Neuromodulation*. 2014;17:665-669; discussion 669.
78 Schu S, Slotty PJ, Bara G, von Knop M, Edgar D, Vesper J. A prospective, randomised, double-blind, placebo-controlled study to examine the effectiveness of burst spinal cord stimulation patterns for the treatment of failed back surgery syndrome. *Neuromodulation*. 2014;17:443-450.
79 Eldabe S, Burger K, Moser H, et al. Dorsal Root Ganglion (DRG) Stimulation in the Treatment of Phantom Limb Pain (PLP). *Neuromodulation*. 2015;18:610-617.

80. Deer TR, Levy RM, Kramer J, et al. Dorsal root ganglion stimulation yielded higher treatment success rate for complex regional pain syndrome and causalgia at 3 and 12 months: a randomized comparative trial. *Pain*. 2017;158:669-681.
81. Kramer J, Liem L, Russo M, Smet I, Van Buyten JP, Huygen F. Lack of body positional effects on paresthesias when stimulating the dorsal root ganglion (DRG) in the treatment of chronic pain. *Neuromodulation*. 2015;18:50-57; discussion 57.
82. Kim C, Ward S, Tomiya A, al. e. Microarchitecture studies of the human multifidus muscle reveal its unique design as a major dynamic stabilizer of the lumbar spine. *54th Annual Meeting of the Orthopaedic Research Society.* , Vol. 1616. Rosemont, Ilinois: Orthopedic Research Society; 2008.
83. Wilke HJ, Wolf S, Claes LE, Arand M, Wiesend A. Stability increase of the lumbar spine with different muscle groups. A biomechanical in vitro study. *Spine (Phila Pa 1976)*. 1995;20:192-198.
84. MacDonald DA, Moseley GL, Hodges PW. The lumbar multifidus: does the evidence support clinical beliefs? *Man Ther*. 2006;11:254-263.
85. Macintosh JE, Valencia F, Bogduk N, Munro RR. The morphology of the human lumbar multifidus. *Clinical biomechanics*. 1986;1:196-204.
86. Hopkins J, Ingersoll C. Arthrogenic muscle inhibition: a limiting factor in joint rehabilitation. . *J Sport Rehabil*. 2009;9.
87. Colloca CJ, Keller TS, Moore RJ, Gunzburg R, Harrison DE. Effects of disc degeneration on neurophysiological responses during dorsoventral mechanical excitation of the ovine lumbar spine. *J Electromyogr Kinesiol*. 2008;18:829-837.
88. Hodges P, Holm AK, Hansson T, Holm S. Rapid atrophy of the lumbar multifidus follows experimental disc or nerve root injury. *Spine (Phila Pa 1976)*. 2006;31:2926-2933.
89. Deckers K, De Smedt K, van Buyten JP, et al. Chronic Low Back Pain: Restoration of Dynamic Stability. *Neuromodulation*. 2015;18:478-486; discussion 486.

We start with the direct stimulation of the Gasserian ganglion.

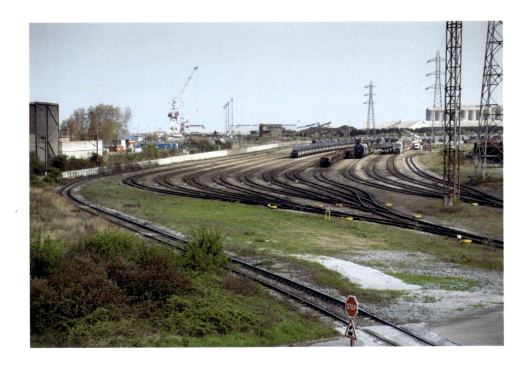

Chapter 2:
Chronic Stimulation of the Gasserian Ganglion in Patients with Trigeminal Neuropathy: A Case Series

Jean-Pierre Van Buyten[1] & Caroline Hens [1]

1 Multidisciplinary Pain Center, AZ Nikolaas, Sint Niklaas, Belgium

Abstract

Between 2009 and 2011 we implanted 8 patients with refractory Trigeminal Neuropathic Pain (TNP) with a custom, tined, percutaneous, tripolar electrode to stimulate the Gasserian Ganglion (TGS). The electrode was positioned with the help of a three-dimensional (3D), real-time, tip-tracked, electromagnetic (EM) guidance system. This technique reduced operating time, and augmented electrode targeting and procedural safety. Six of the eight patients had pain relief of at least 30%, all significantly tapered medication-intake (4 stopped opioids completely), two had minor dislocations, and none suffered any major complication. This EM stimulation technique is a valuable, reversible, minimally invasive method to treat refractory TNP.

Keywords:
Facial neuropathic pain, trigeminal ganglion, percutaneous stimulation, and electromagnetic guidance

Introduction

Craniofacial pain is a complex group of clinical conditions that are difficult to diagnose. In the past, pain occurring in the distribution of the trigeminal nerve often led to the diagnosis of trigeminal neuralgia (TN), whereas the diagnosis of trigeminal neuropathic pain (TNP) may have been more accurate. Subsequently various TN therapies, including high dose anticonvulsants, neuroleptics, tricyclic antidepressants, and opioids, as well as microvascular decompression and neurodestructive procedures of the trigeminal nerve were often applied for TNP with poor results. In fact, Sweet's review of TNP showed that 73% of patients that underwent TN type neurodestructive procedures failed to obtain relief, and many were actually worse.[1] In order to facilitate a correct diagnosis of craniofacial pain, Burchiel proposed a classification scheme based on the patients' symptoms and history.[2] (Figure 1).

Pain category	History/Pain pattern	Other names
Trigeminal Neuralgia type 1	Spontaneous onset (>50% episodic pain)	Idiopathic Trigeminal Neuralgia
Trigeminal Neuralgia type 2	Spontaneous onset (≥50% constant pain)	Atypical Trigeminal Neuralgia
Trigeminal Neuropathic pain	Trigeminal injury - unintentional (trauma,	
Trigeminal Deafferentation pain	Trigeminal injury – intentional deafferentation (after destructive	Anesthesia Dolorosa/Hypoesthesia
Symptomatic Trigeminal Neuralgia/MS	Multiple Sclerosis	
Symptomatic Trigeminal Neuralgia/other	Posterior fossa mass lesions, Chiari mal-formation	Secondary Trigeminal Neuralgia
Post herpetic Neuralgia	Trigeminal Herpes zoster outbreak	
Atypical facial pain	Somatoform pain disorder	

Figure 1: Classification of Craniofacial Pain by Burchiel (2003)[2]

In this classification, Type I presents as spontaneous onset of paroxysmal facial pain, whereas Type II is predominantly constant. Patients describe their symptoms as a constant burning sensation, often associated with allodynia, hyperpathia and dysesthesia.

We distinguish TNP as trigeminal neuropathy caused by injury to the trigeminal system (e.g. trauma, dental/ sinus procedures, craniofacial surgery); trigeminal deafferentation pain (TDP) as following procedures treating TN (e.g. peripheral nerve ablation, Radiofrequency (RF) Gasserian Ganglion lesioning); and post herpetic neuralgia (PHN) following herpes zoster infection.

Sheldon first attempted electrical stimulation of the Trigeminal Gasserian Ganglion (TGS) in 1967.[3] In 1977, Meyerson and Hákanson sutured a bipolar plate electrode to the dura overlying the trigeminal ganglion using an open craniotomy technique.[4] However this was abandoned due to the risks involving craniotomy, and the impossibility of testing the stimulation parameters during placement. In 1984, Meglio and Steude described the first percutaneous technique.[5,6] In a large implant series, Steude concluded that 86% of patients with TNP, and 100% of patients with TDP had relief.[7,8] He also noted that PHN did not respond well. Tasker's group reported similar results.[9]

Although complications were rare, the most common problem historically was electrode dislocation due to the unique anatomy of the foramen ovale. 10, 11 Thus, several shapes and sizes of electrodes were used to try to overcome this problem including a sigma-electrode, quinta-trigeminal anchored electrode, and a sacral nerve root stimulation electrode (Medtronic Neurological Pisces #3483 sizes 0.7mm, 0.9mm, 1.2mm, Minneapolis, Minnesota). The larger electrodes initially seemed to dislocate less, but elicited dysesthesia. 10 Mehrkens and Steude even noted that the specially shaped sigma electrode dislocated in nearly 100% of patients.[10]

Thus, with a focus on improving anatomic targeting and reducing electrode migration, we performed a series of TGS in 8 patients with TNP using a 3D, real- time, tip-tracked EM guidance system with intraoperative CT Scan (The O-arm® Surgical Imaging Stealth Station®, Medtronic Surgical Navigation Technologies, Minneapolis, Minnesota) and a new custom tined electrode

Methods

This retrospective chart review did not require ethical committee approval. Eight patients with refractory TNP were included in this series between 2009-2011. Diagnosis was based on clinical examination and medical history. All patients except one (case 6) had iatrogenic TNP. All patients had exhausted treatment with a variety of pharmacological agents (tricyclic antidepressants, neuroleptics, anticonvulsants, opioids) without any significant relief. Most had one or more peripheral nerve blocks or neurodestructive procedures in the area of the trigeminal ganglion. Two patients previously had a motor cortex stimulation implant without improvement (Figure 2).

A detailed evaluation by our pain psychologist was performed to screen for psychological contraindications to implant. As well, psychosocial stressors (e.g. major depression, anxiety, fear, personality disorders) were assessed in order to optimize the result of therapy. Helping patients build realistic expectations regarding the TGS implant, and to learn how to cope with any residual pain was considered a valuable preoperative contribution.

Surgical technique

All patients underwent a trial for at least 4 weeks with an externalized electrode. On the day prior to implant, a 3D-CTScan of the head was constructed which would be used to guide needle placement into the foramen ovale using the O-arm® EM neuro-navigational system. In the operating room the patient was placed in supine position on a carbon table. After installing standard monitoring, sedation was given using propofol (Diprivan®, AstraZeneca, Wilmington, DE). The O-arm® was placed around the head of the patient, along with a fluoroscope, allowing both x-ray and 3D-reconstruction needle localization. Based on the 3D-images, entry-and target points were set and a virtual track proposed in axonal, coronal and sagittal views (Figure 3).

A local anesthetic was then injected at the entry zone. A small incision was made lateral to the labial commissure, and a 15-gauge needle inserted. All incisions were made by the plastic surgeon at our center to obtain the most aesthetic result after wound healing.

The needle was then guided by 3D real-time, EM tip tracking into the foramen ovale. Under continuous fluoroscopy the electrode was inserted until the tip reached the clivus. At that moment the patient was awakened, and a test-stimulation performed until paresthesia was evoked in the area of the neuropathy. The needle was withdrawn under continuous fluoroscopy to assure maintenance of the electrode in the correct position, and a Marceline 4-0 suture placed on the electrode at the entry site. No anchor was used. The patient was then re-sedated and the electrode tunneled subcutaneously between the maxilla and mandibular region. A second suture was then placed in a pre-auricular position. We chose this position to prevent traction on the lead by movement of the neck and jaw. Finally, after a positive trial, an internal pulse generator (Medtronic Itrel III, Minneapolis, Minnesota) was placed in the supraclavicular fossa. Skull-base X-ray and CT scan confirmation films were obtained (Figure 4).

Case	Age/Gender	Etiology	Area of pain	Previous treatments	Result of stimulation	Last follow visit
1: DJ	F 74Y	Maxillofacial surgery	V1-2	-Gabapentin, Opioids, TCA's -RF Gasserian Ganglion -Thalamic stimulation	+ 50% relief	6 months
2: OS	F 66Y	Excision glandular tumor	V1-2-3	-Opioids, Gabapentin -RF Gasserian Ganglion -PRF Facial Nerve	+ 40% relief	6 months
3: DWI	F 37Y	Post trauma	V2	-Opioids, TCA's, Anti-epileptics -Gamma knife -Vascular decompression (Janetta)	+ 30% relief	5 months
4: PL	M 62Y	Unknown	V2-3	-Gabapentin, opioids, TCA's, Carbamazepine -Infiltration Gasserian and Sphenopalatine Ganglion -Motor Cortex Stimulation (MCS)	50-60% initial MCS x 5 years, now 40-50% relief with TGS	2 months
5: VM	F 70Y	Herpes zoster infection	V1-2-3	-Opioids, TCA's, Anti-epileptics -RF Gasserian and Sphenopalatine Ganglion -Occipital stimulation -RF C2	V1 50% V2-3 20%	2 months
6: PE	F 47Y	Excision parotid gland	V2-3	-Opioids, Rivotril, TCA's, Pregabaline, Gabapentin -RF Sphenopalatine Ganglion -Occipital stimulation	Displacement electrode	Revision
7: VDA	F 70Y	Unknown	V3	-Gabapentin, opioids, TCA's, Carbamazepine -Dental extractions -RF Gasserian Ganglion -Motor Cortex Stimulation (MCS)	Displacement electrode	Revision
8: LMT	F 72Y	Intervention for essential trigeminal neuralgia, vascular decompression, and RF Gasserian	V1,2,3	-Gabapentin, opioids, TCA's, Carbamazepine, SNRI's -Vascular decompression (Janetta)	+ 80% pain relief	1 month

Figure 2: Patient population, etiology, and results of stimulation.

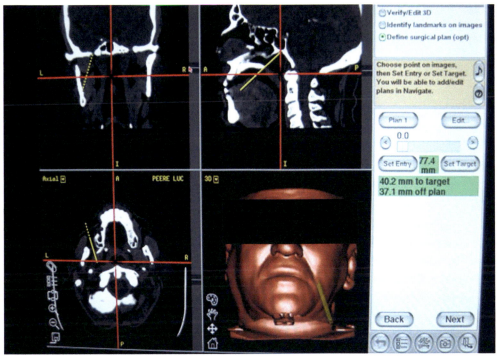

Figure 3: Real time electromagnetic guidance (EM) view.

Given the history of dislodgement, a new curved, tined; tripolar electrode design (Medtronic Neurological, Minneapolis, Minnesota, Model 09053) was applied in these cases to limit retraction and displacement (Figure 5). In comparison to former foramen ovale electrodes, this design is more flexible after removal of the guide- wire, reducing traction or irritation with movement of the head and face. As noted by Mehrkens and Steude[10] a 1.2mm diameter electrode was chosen to prevent dysesthesia. As well, as specific anchoring devices had not reduced the risk of dislodgement (and could create facial area irritation), Marceline sutures were used to fix the electrode subcutaneously at the mandibular and pre-auricular region

For our patients, the most comfortable frequency of stimulation was 50Hertz. Pulse-width initially was programmed at 450msec. The amplitude of the stimulus varied between 0.2V and 2.5 volts. Higher amplitudes tend to activate the masseter muscle or the periorbital muscles giving rise to blurred vision and visible contractions of the jaw. Since low voltages were applied, battery longevity is expected.

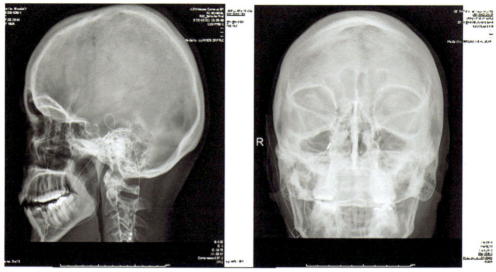

Figure 4: Lateral and frontal fluoroscopic image of TGS electrode.

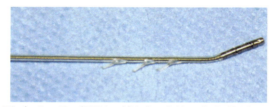

Figure 5: Custom-made Tripolar Bent Tined TGS Lead (Medtronic Neurological®, Minneapolis, Minnesota, Model 09053).

Results

In this series, there were seven females and one male with refractory TNP. Our psychologist screened all patients before test stimulation was performed. There was a hesitation for 1 patient (case 3) that showed some psychiatric history. The origin of the pain was due to surgery or trauma in 4 cases, neuropathy following interventional procedures for TN in 2 cases, and unknown in 2 cases. All the patients had pain relief of at least 30% during the test period, and requested and received a definitive implant. There were no major surgical complications. There was no worsening by this procedure in any patient. This flexible and small electrode elicited no uncomfortable dysesthesia. In two cases the electrode showed a minor dislodgement with altering of the pain relief and paresthesia. Both were revised easily under fluoroscopic guidance. In one (case 3) the electrode had eroded into the buccal mucosa, but showed no infection. Post stimulation, all patients were able to taper down significantly on their opioids, with 4 patients stopping them completely.

Conclusion

Trigeminal Neuropathy (TNP) is one of a number of complex craniofacial pain syndromes. Differentiating it clinically from TN is crucial as neurodestructive procedures could worsen TNP. From 2009-2011 we performed TGS in 8 patients with refractory TNP using a 3D, real-time, tip-tracked, electromagnetic (EM) guidance system. Six of the eight patients have had stable electrode placement with pain relief of at least 30%. This technique was a valuable, precise, minimally invasive method that reduced operating room time and created no major com- plications. Further large-scale, long-term studies should be performed.

References

1   Sweet WH. Percutaneous methods for the treatment of trigeminal neuralgia and other faciocephalic pain; comparison with microvascular decompression. *Semin Neurol*. 1988;8:272-279.

2   Burchiel KJ. A new classification for facial pain. *Neurosurgery*. 2003;53:1164-1166; discussion 1166-1167.

3   Shelden CH, Pudenz RH, Doyle J. Electrical control of facial pain. *Am J Surg*. 1967;114:209-212.

4   Meyerson BA, Hakanson S. Suppression of pain in trigeminal neuropathy by electric stimulation of the gasserian ganglion. *Neurosurgery*. 1986;18:59-66.

5   Meglio M. Percutaneous implantable chronic electrode for radiofrequency stimulation of the gasserian ganglion: a perspective in the management of trigeminal pain. *Acta Neurochir (Wien)*. 1984:521-525.

6   Steude U. Radiofrequency electrical stimulation of the Gasserian ganglion in patients with atypical trigeminal pain: methods of percutaneous temporaty test-stimulation and permanent implantation of stimulation devices. *Acta Neurochir (Wien)*. 1984;Suppl 33:481-486.

7   Steude U. Chronic trigeminal nerve stimulation for the relief of persistent pain. In: Gildenberg P, Tasker R, eds. *Textbook of Stereotactic and Functional Neurosurgery*. New York: McGraw-Hill; 1998. 1557–1564.

8   Steude U. Percutaneous electrical stimulation of the Gasserian ganglion in patients with atypical trigeminal neuralgia. *The Pain Clinic*. 1985:239.

9   Taub E, Munz M, Tasker RR. Chronic electrical stimulation of the gasserian ganglion for the relief of pain in a series of 34 patients. *J Neurosurg*. 1997;86:197-202.

10   Mehrkens JH, Steude U. Chronic electrostimulation of the trigeminal ganglion in trigeminal neuropathy: current state and future prospects. *Acta Neurochir Suppl*. 2007;97:91-97.

11   Osenbach R. Neurostimulation for the Treatment of Intractable Facial Pain *Pain Medicine*. 2006;7.

We analyzed the predictive value of a positive trial and other parameters that determine a successful outcome.

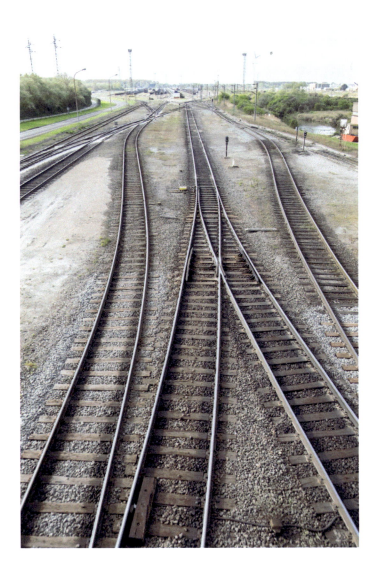

Chapter 3
Stimulation of the Gasserian ganglion in the treatment of refractory trigeminal neuropathy

Lise Kustermans [1]; Jean-Pierre Van Buyten[2], Iris Smet [2], Wim Coucke [3], Constantinus Politis [1]

[1] Department of Oral and Maxillofacial Surgery, University Hospital Leuven, Belgium
[2] Department of Anesthesia and Pain Management, AZ Nikolaas, Sint-Niklaas, Belgium
[3] Department of Oral and Maxillofacial Surgery-IMPATH, KULeuven, Heverlee, Belgium

Journal of Cranio-Maxillo-Facial Surgery. 201; 45: 39-46

Abstract

Objectives: We evaluated the effectiveness of a custom-made neurostimulator with which to treat patients for refractory trigeminal neuropathic pain (TNP) at the level of the Gasserian ganglion.

Materials and Methods: A retrospective analysis of 22 patients referred to our pain clinic, AZ Sint- Nikolaas, between 2010 and 2015, was conducted using the McGill Pain and EuroQoL questionnaire before, two weeks after, and at the final follow-up after neurostimulator treatment.

Results: Successful test stimulations were achieved for 77.3% of patients, with satisfactory long-term pain relief reported by 44% at 24 months. The predictive value of the trial stimulation was 80%, with 82.4% of patients reporting one or more complication, the most common being neck discomfort due to fibrosis. A small cohort size (n=22) limited our statistical analyses. However younger patients presented with a higher incidence of negative results after 24 months or physical complications. Cut-off ages were set at the age of 62 and 58 years respectively.

Conclusion: Stimulation of the Gasserian ganglion is a promising technique for the treatment of refractory TNP and should be considered ahead of more invasive techniques such as motor cortex or deep brain stimulation. The referral of refractory TNP patients should also be accomplished as early as possible to improve outcome.

Keywords:
Trigeminal neuropathic pain; Neurostimulation; Gasserian ganglion; Intractable pain; Persistent postoperative pain

Introduction

Craniofacial pain has a wide array of possible underlying etiologies. A commonly used classification for facial pain proposed by Burchiel [1] (Table1) is based on the patient's symptoms and history. This study focuses on a subgroup of patients that suffer from neuropathic craniofacial pain caused by a lesion on the trigeminal nerve, either following an accidental non-intentional injury (e.g. external trauma, dental procedures), a herpes zoster infection, or as the result of an invasive ablative procedure alongside its tract (trigeminal deafferentation pain).

In cases of (peripheral) trigeminal neuropathic pain (TNP), tricyclic antidepressants, and/or anticonvulsive drugs remain the treatments of choice [2]. For this group of patients, in comparison to classic trigeminal neuralgia (cTN), pharmacological intervention is often unsatisfactory with patients' becoming tolerant to drugs while at the same time being susceptible to their potent and unpleasant side effects. According to many previous studies, the initial success rates for this approach are estimated to be about 50% [3, 4]. For pharmacologically refractory TNP, the indications for surgical treatment such as microvascular decompression and neurodestructive interventions (e.g. radiofrequency, gamma knife procedure) remain unclear. Alongside many other published studies Sweet [5] showed that neurodestructive procedures conferred no beneficial effects, and instead aggravated the condition for almost three quarters (73%) of all patients [5-9]. We feel that these patients, enduring persistent neuropathic pain, might instead benefit from neuromodulation techniques. Given the considerable level of suffering for this cohort, together with the societal burden imposed by the costs of chronic care, and absence from work, we believe that our new approach to neuromodulation using a custom- made neurostimulator (NS) at the level of the Gasserian ganglion (GG), may be of benefit.

Table 1: Burchiel's classification of facial pain syndromes[1, 9, 10].

Diagnosis	History	Causes
Spontaneous onset		
TN, type I	>50% paroxysmal pain	Neurovascular compression of trigeminal nerve or unknown
TN, type II	<50% paroxysmal pain	Neurovascular compression of trigeminal nerve or unknown
Symptomatic TN	TN due to multiple sclerosis	Demyelination
Atypical facial pain	Somatoform pain disorder	
Peripheral trigeminal injury		
TNP	Incidental non-intentional injury	ENT/oral surgery, facial trauma, stroke, etc.
TDP	Trigeminal injury from peripheral ablation	RF rhizotomy, glycerol rhizolysis, GKR, balloon compression, etc.
Postherpetic neuralgia (PHN)	Herpes zoster outbreak	Shingles involving trigeminal distribution

TN = trigeminal neuralgia; AFP = atypical facial pain; TNP = trigeminal neuropathic pain; TDP= trigeminal deafferentation pain; ENT = ear, nose and throat; RF = radiofrequency (nowadays selective thermolesion); GKR = gamma-knife radiosurgery.

Several studies have been conducted concerning the efficacy of this type of approach, although, until now, they have generally included small patient cohorts, with no contemporary reports available. Meyerson and Hakansson[8] were the first to demonstrate a successful outcome, with 11 of 14 patients reporting a significant reduction of pain after a follow-up of 4 years and more.[8] In their large-scale study (235 patients with a follow-up ≥ 5 years; 1980-2005), Mehrkens and Steude [7] reported that 52% of patients considered that their pain was halved.[9] A large cohort studied in 2001 3, including data from eight clinical studies involving 267 patients, concluded that 48% of the 233 patients showing pharmacological refractory trigeminal neuropathy, demonstrated pain reduction of more than 50% during a long-term observation period (from 6 months to 15 years). An initial four-week trial stimulation appeared to be an effective way to stratify patients that might respond well to this treatment modality, and were found to be suitable for the implantation of a pulse generator in the infraclavicular region. It was reported that 83% and 79% of all patients with positive test stimulations experienced, respectively, long-term pain reduction in excess of 50% and 75%[3]. This agrees with the findings of Mehrkens and Steude [7], who identified good-to-excellent analgesia in 82% of patients after permanent implantation following a positive trial stimulation period. [7] However, the reported incidence of positive test results varied significantly among the different studies, ranging from 47% to 80%. [3]

In contrast to an electrode designed for deep brain stimulation (DBS), or the 8-pole electrode used for spinal cord stimulation (SCS), which is in widespread use and has been extensively applied for decades, an electrode adequately adjusted to the small dimension of the GG is not yet commercially available. In their study, Meyerson and Hakansson [8] used a bipolar plate, sutured to the dura overlying the GG, using an open craniotomy technique. This high-risk approach was subsequently abandoned. [8] Mehrkens and Steude[7] described the first percutaneous technique for GG stimulation, but they still experienced a high incidence of electrode dislocation due to the unique anatomy of the foramen ovale. [7] For this reason we developed a custom-made tripolar, bent, tined TGS lead (Model 09053) in collaboration with Medtronic (Figure 1). In this study, we retrospectively analyzed data from 22 patients to evaluate the overall success rate achieved with our custom-made electrode, with real-time 3D electromagnetic navigation system for electrode positioning at the level of the GG.

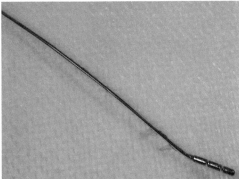

Figure 1: Custom-made, tripolar, bent, tined TGS lead (Model 09053), developed in collaboration with Medtronic.

Any trial therapeutic modality for this patient subset raises questions about the profile of these patients, the success rate of neurostimulation, the predictive value of a positive trial for long- term success, and other parameters that determine a successful outcome. We wished to address these issues, as well as examining the complication rate and type associated with this procedure.

Materials and methods

We included all patients referred to the pain clinic AZ Sint-Nikolaas, Sint-Niklaas, with refractory neuropathic pain, who had been implanted (between 2010 and 2015) with an NS electrode at the level of the GG. Because this procedure is part of our standard therapeutic arsenal and the retrospective character of this study, no approval of the ethical committee was required. These patients were implanted with a custom- made tripolar, bent, tined TGS Lead, developed in collaboration with Medtronic (Figure 1). The electrode tip depicts a slightly bent design that facilitates contact with the GG, just beyond the foramen ovale. The tip is also equipped with two tines for attachment at the level of the foramen ovale, which reduces the possibility of dislocation as demonstrated by an older generation NS, without tines, which was dislodged in the single patient who received this implant

(2005). In 2011, we implanted a tined lead into this patient; only data from this lead were analyzed in this study.

The procedure itself is performed in two stages. The first is a trial of at least 4 weeks' duration with an externalized electrode. On the day prior to implantation, a 3D computed tomography (CT) scan of the head is obtained and transferred to the neuronavigation machine, used to guide the needle into the foramen ovale. In the operating room the patient is placed in the supine position on a radiolucent table. The patient is informed about and prepared for a wake-up procedure to ensure proper placement of the electrode, afterwards insertion is performed under sedation using propofol. The O-arm is placed around the head of the patient, allowing continuous high-definition fluoroscopy and perioperative CT imaging with 3D reconstruction. For lead placement, electro-magnetic neuronavigation technology (Medtronic Stealth Station) based on the preoperative multislice CT-scan and 3D reconstruction was used. The head of the patient is positioned in a magnetic field, using a strong magnet attached to the operating room table. Entry and target points are defined on the stealth station, generating a virtual track for the placement of the needle into the foramen ovale. This track can be followed in the axial, sagittal, and coronal planes. A local anesthetic is then injected at the entry point. A small incision is made lateral to the labial commissure, and a 15-gauge needle inserted. The needle is then guided by 3D real-time electromagnetic tip tracking into the foramen ovale, following the track indicated by the Stealth Station. Once the needle is in place (entering the skull base), the electrode is inserted through the needle under continuous fluoroscopy until its tip reaches the clivus. At that moment the patient is awakened, and a test stimulation using low twitches at 2 Hz performed until paresthesia (and subtle facial muscle twitching) is evoked in the area of neuropathic pain. The needle is withdrawn under continuous fluoroscopic control to ensure that the electrode remains in the correct position, and a non-absorbable braided 4-0 suture (Mersilene; Ethicon, Somerville, N.J., USA) is placed on the electrode at the entry site. The patient is then re-sedated and the electrode tunneled subcutaneously along the neck to the infra- clavicular region. Finally, in case of a positive trial, an internal pulse generator (IPG) (Itrel 3, Itrel, Medtronic) is placed in the infraclavicular fossa. Skull-base X-ray and CT scan confirmation films are subsequently obtained.

Retrospective analyses of medical files were conducted for all patients. Only 4 patients completed the McGill Pain Questionnaire prior to implantation and at about 2 weeks after implantation, when wound healing was complete. Subsequently, between December 2015 and January 2016, we contacted every patient by telephone to repeat the McGill Pain and EuroQoL questionnaire in a retrospective manner, collecting data for the moments before placement, 2 weeks after, and at the time of final recall. Where discrepancies arose in pain description during the call, compared to prior data collection, we chose to work with the original dataset to prevent under-reporting of temporary clinical improvements. During our study timeline, 2 patients committed suicide because they failed to experience long-term pain relief by this, or any other technique. Pain scores for one of these patients could be derived from data in his medical file, corroborated by phone interviews with relatives. For the other patient, there were no pain level data reported, so this patient was ultimately excluded from the study. A third patient requested euthanasia for the same reason.

While processing the data, we defined outcomes at 6 and 24 months of follow-up. A "successful" outcome was recorded when the following criteria were met:
- Final implantation of an implantable pulse generator following a positive test stimulation.
- Pain levels not rated as "severe" or "extremely severe", based on patient feedback using visual analogue scores (VAS) in the McGill Pain questionnaire.
- AND reduction of the number and/or dose of pain medication.

- AND/OR improvement of sleep patterns (McGill Pain questionnaire).
- AND no major complications leading to removal of the electrode.

All data were analyzed using S-Plus 8.0 for Linux (Tibco, Palo Alto, CA, USA). Differences in McGill scores between time points were assessed by a paired Wilcoxon test. Relations between risk factors and outcome variables were first assessed by generalized linear models. A stepwise regression model selection was applied to find the subset of risk factors that have the strongest association with each of the outcome variables. We obtained an age cut-off that determined the greatest risk of an adverse outcome using ROC- curve analyses. In addition, a Kaplan-Meier analysis was performed to model the evolution of pain relief over time.

Results

Patient characteristics

The procedure of GG NS insertion was first introduced at our clinic in 2010. Since then, 22 patients have been implanted with an electrode, with 9 procedures completed in 2011. Our patient cohort included a predominance of female patients (16/22), with interventions occurring from ages 32-76 years, with an average age of 59. Eight patients were referred from another pain clinic to our center, 12 patients were from the department of neurology or neurosurgery. 1 patient presented at her own initiative having heard about our new neuromodulation technique on television. The data from one deceased patient was missing. None of these patients had been referred by either their general practitioner or dentist. 77% of our cohort had suffered with TNP for at least 5 years before NS therapy (range 0.5-16 years, average 8 years). In nearly half of the patients, only one branch of the trigeminal nerve was affected. For the remainder, there was involvement of V2 + V3, or V1 + V2 + V3. An equivalent number of patients were affected on the left versus right side of the face. In 82% (18/22) of cases, the etiology of the TNP was iatrogenic, due to a peripheral surgical intervention in 55% (e.g. implant placement, tooth extraction), or a central surgical or ablative intervention in 45%. 10 of 22 patients (45%) also suffered from one or more coexisting pain syndromes such as anesthesia dolorosa (n = 2), cluster headache (n = 2), migraine (n = 1), (former) classic trigeminal neuralgia (n = 6), or a generalized pain syndrome like fibromyalgia, chronic fatigue syndrome, or polymyalgia rheumatica (n = 2). Nearly all patients (95%) had undergone pharmacological treatment with anti-epileptics and/or antidepressants without satisfactory and/or lasting pain relief (Fig. 2). At least 77% had tried 3 or more classes of pain medication, with 45% using 6 or more, 32%, 7 or more, and 18%, 8 or more. Three quarters (73%) had undergone a previous ablative procedure at the level of the GG as a treatment modality (Fig. 3). With 55% of our population on retirement, 36% on invalidity, and 9% actively working, we find that 80% of work-entitled patients are reduced to invalidity. Almost two thirds of patients demonstrated a history of, and/or a present major mood or anxiety disorder. About half of the patients smoke, drink alcohol, and/or exhibit excessive drug abuse.

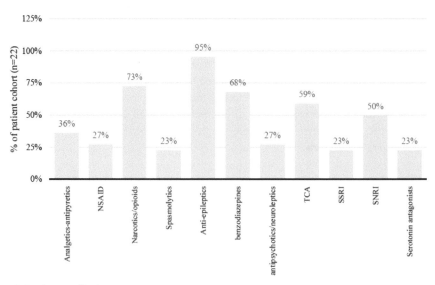

Figure 2: Previous medication.

Outcome

Success at test stimulation (followed by definitive implantation of an IPG) occurred for 17 of 22 patients (77.3%). A criterion for concluding a positive test result was any subjective pain reduction given that these patients had no alternative treatment left to pursue. A positive result is also cost-effective, given the 10-year life- span of the battery being implanted. The majority of the patients with a positive test result (88%, 15/17 patients) reported pain reduction of at least 50% after placement of a permanent implant; two patients reported inferior pain reductions of 44% and 33%.

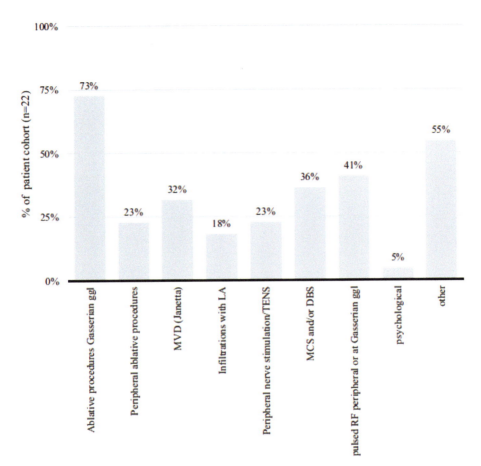

Figure 3: Previous treatment.

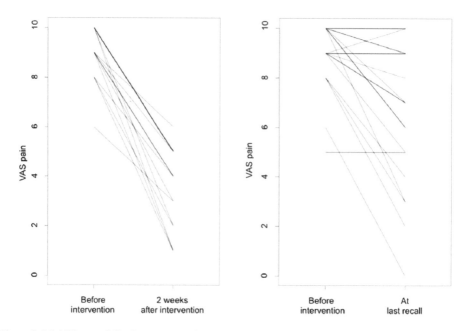

Figure 4: Pain VAS-score following neurostimulation intervention (left n=16 and right n=21).

Figure 4 shows the evolution of the individual VAS-scores just before stimulation, 2 weeks after intervention, and at the time of last recall, with 0/10 indicating no pain and 10/10 the worst imaginary pain. The average VAS-score in the overall patient cohort, and in the positive trial subgroup before intervention was 9/ 10 (ranging from 6 to 10/10). The average VAS-score in the positive trial group at the moment of last recall was still 7/10 (ranging from 0 to 10/10) although reduction to 4/10 (ranging 1-6/10) was initially achieved 2 weeks after intervention. This means an average VAS-score decrease of 5/10 and 2/10 over the short- and long-term respectively. In other words, the original average VAS-score is reduced by 61% (ranging 33-90%) two weeks after intervention, but only by 29% (ranging -11% to 100%) at last recall. These data illustrate a partial relapse following a substantial initial benefit. However, VAS-scores 2 weeks after intervention, and at last recall, appear to differ significantly from the initial VAS-scores (p-values 0.0004 and 0.00021 respectively; Table 2), indicating a long-term significant benefit in terms of pain level. When observing each patient individually, 9/16 (56%) reported no remaining benefit (long-term), 2/16 (13%) reported a partial increase in pain, and 5/16 (31%) reported permanent pain reduction. Of more significance may be the improvement observed regarding the "quality" of the pain. Initially, all patients described their pain as either "severe" (25%) or "extremely severe" (75%). Immediately after intervention, there were no reports of extremely severe pain, with only 1 patient describing severe pain (no patients were pain free). At last recall, 44% of patients were reporting neither "extremely severe" nor "severe" pain levels. One patient even reported being pain free (Figure 5). When taking into account the follow-up period after intervention, there are some caveats to our conclusions. The observational period ranged from only 4.5 months to 63 months (mean of 43 months, when taking into account the last recall time or time of death), for which two patients failed to reach the 2 year-cut off. A survival analysis (Figure 6) shows that of the 17 patients with a positive test stimulation who proceeded to definitive implantation:

(i) 7 (41.2%) have yet to experience a total loss of beneficial effect.
(ii) There were no relapses during the first 6 months after intervention.
(iii) Where relapse occurred, in 80% (8/10) of cases it arose be- tween 6 and 24 months of follow-up.
(iv) The chance of experiencing long-term pain reduction after 24 months is 45.7%.

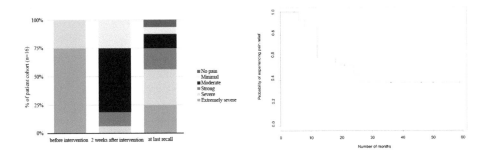

Figure 5: McGill description of pain.   Figure 6: Survival analyses (Kaplan-Meier; n=17).

With one patient failing to reach the 6-month follow-up threshold, and a second failing to reach the 24-month threshold, the success rate at 6 months of follow-up was 93.8% (15/16), decreasing to 46.7% (i.e. some beneficial effects from NS; 7/15) at 24 months' follow-up.

The burden on quality of life with pain disorders is significant and is important to take into account when evaluating the efficacy of a treatment modality. Given the high level of analgesics used by this population, it was remarkable that only 2 of 17 (12%) subjects were not able to partially or completely stop their medication use after initiation of the stimulation therapy. Two patients stopped using pain medication altogether. Additionally, intolerance to pain medication had already resulted in two patients curtailing medication use 6 months before the stimulation intervention. In parallel to the significant improvements observed with the pain VAS-scores (Table 2), the beneficial effects on daily and social activity were significant and permanent (p-value 0.0059 and 0.0145 respectively). Substantial early improvements in sleep quality with that fraction of patients rating their sleep as "good" increased from 30% to 67% (nobody mentioned "excellent" sleep patterns; p = 0.0022). However, this early improvement was again eroded by the last follow-up (40%, p = 0.6561). The pro- portion of patients reporting rarely, or never being woken by pain at night, also improved from 40% to 87% early after intervention. However, these data must be interpreted with caution given that more than half of our population (57%) were prescribed sleep medication. When questioning the need to lie down to rest during daytime, a similar loss of improvement was observed long-term (p = 0.1258).

Table 2: Effect of neurostimulation on McGill Pain Scores.

Outcome	Difference	p-Value
VAS pain	2 weeks after – before intervention	0.0004
VAS pain	At last recall – before intervention	0.0021
EuroQol score	2 weeks after – before intervention	0.0019
EuroQol score	At last recall – before intervention	0.3017
VAS daily activity	2 weeks after – before intervention	0.0023
VAS daily activity	At last recall – before intervention	0.0059
VAS social activity	2 weeks after – before intervention	0.0008
VAS social activity	At last recall – before intervention	0.0145
VAS resting need	2 weeks after – before intervention	0.0023
VAS resting need	At last recall – before intervention	0.1258
VAS sleep quality	2 weeks after – before intervention	0.0022
VAS sleep quality	At last recall – before intervention	0.6561

Subjective health scores (0/100 representing a very poor state of health, 100/100, being excellent) were 32/100 (30-90) for the patient group upon presentation at our clinic. Following stimulation treatment, this rose to 66/100 (30-90), representing a significant improvement (p ¼ 0.0019), before declining to 42/100 (0e90) on last recall (p ¼ 0.3017). The high incidence of complications may have contributed to this relapse (Table 3). Although no major complications necessitating removal of the device (e.g. serious infections), only 18% of patients reported no unpleasant adverse event. The most frequent complaint was some discomfort at the level of the neck due to fibrotic tissue at the connection of the electrode lead and extension. Uncomplicated local infections that could be managed conservatively, without removal of the stimulator, arose for three patients. With one patient, an abdominal skin infection occurred at the in-situ pulse generator, which had already been implanted for previous lumbar stimulation. Intra-oral erosion with perforation of the oral mucosa also occurred relatively frequently, particularly for 4 patients (24%). Although this phenomenon did not influence outcome negatively, the patients in question were always greatly upset by this complication and often requested treatment revision thereafter.

Table 3: Complication rate (n = 17).

Complication	Number of patients (n = 17) (%)
Intra-oral erosion	4 (24%)
Dislocation of lead	2 (12%)
Major infection (e.g. meningitis, sepsis,...)	0 (0%)
Uncomplicated local infection (conservatively managed without removal of stimulator)	3 (18%)
Mechanical defect (e.g. leakage of lead, remote control, replacement battery,...)	4 (24%)
Dysesthesia and/or physical discomfort (e.g. muscle cramps, fibrosis connection neck,...)	7 (41%)
Incapability of patient to understand and adjust settings	3 (18%)
None	3 (18%)

An important complicating aspect of the treatment is the ability of each patient to understand how to manage the remote-control unit, and to adjust the settings of stimulation so as to obtain the best possible results. Unfortunately, this remains a major issue for almost 1/5 of the patient cohort, with stimulation parameters needed to be reset on a regular basis. The adjustment of stimulation characteristics, lead repositioning when displaced, or battery replacement, was not considered as outcomes reflecting the failure of the method itself. We were also unsure as to the need for patients to experience paresthesia, which can be disturbing. Sub-threshold stimulation or high frequency (10 kHz) stimulation without paresthesia might yield equivalent or even superior results, this possibility is still to be explored.

Although risk stratification was carried out to identify those patients at risk of a negative trial stimulation, no useful predictive determinants could be identified. A wide range of variables were taken into account. Concerning outcome after a follow-up of 24 months, 3 variables showed a significant correlation with a negative outcome, a comparatively young age (p = 0.0426), no previous peripheral ablative procedure (p ¼ 0.0401), and no previous peripheral or central pulsed radio frequency treatment (p = 0.018). A cut-off at the age of 62 was set, with only 14.3% of patients obtaining a successful result after 24 months when <62 years old, in comparison to 75% for those 62 years of age or older. To obtain a more reliable result, complications were divided into two groups. The first, defined as physical, included intra-oral erosion, dislocation of the lead, major infection (e.g. sepsis, meningitis), uncomplicated local infection which could be managed conservatively without removal of stimulator, and physical discomfort (e.g. dysesthesia, muscle cramps, fibrosis). The second group included mechanical complications (e.g. high impedance on the lead, problems with the remote control, need for battery replacement) or inability of the patient to understand and adjust stimulation set- tings. A younger age was significantly correlated with a higher incidence of physical complications (p ¼ 0.0051), whereas older patients showed a substantially higher risk of mechanical complications (p ¼ 0.0431). Cut-off ages were set at the age of 58 and 66 years for physical and mechanical complications respectively. The only other risk factors that correlated with the occurrence of a physical complication, besides age, were excessive use of alcohol, smoking, or drugs (p = 0.0018).

Discussion

Stimulation of the GG is a promising technique for the treatment of refractory TNP, and should be attempted before more invasive techniques. A major advantage of this neurostimulation technique is that it does not exacerbate pain, agreeing with a previous report by Mehrkens and Steude. [7] We envisage future use of Gasserian stimulation early in the treatment of neuropathic pain, given the present failure of antidepressants and/or anticonvulsants, or any ablative intervention, to provide long lasting pain relief. At least 77% of our patient cohort had tried 3 or more classes of pain medication, with 45% having attempted 6 or more. 73% had also undergone a previous ablative procedure at the level of the GG, with no sustained effect.

An improved sensitivity to, and awareness of this pain problem, with new therapeutic approaches are necessary, especially for primary care physicians and dentists. Currently, many patients are misdiagnosed, resulting in long delays before receiving appropriate neuromodulation therapy. [4] In our patient population, we observed an average waiting period of 8 years (range 0.5-16 years) before proceeding to neurostimulation, indicating a significant delay, partially due to the lack of an efficient and straightforward treatment algorithm. Although a delay in intervention could not be established as a risk factor for a negative outcome (due to the small cohort size), previous experience from studies on SCS would indicate that this would probably be the case. [6] Previously it has been suggested that waiting lists for assessment by a pain specialist should not exceed 8 weeks, as the efficacy of SCS treatment is time dependent. Success rates exceed 80% if implantation occurs within 2 years of symptom onset, compared with 15% for patients fitted with implants 20 years after the onset of pain. Furthermore, TNP dramatically affects quality of life. Underestimating the severity of this problem, as well as under treatment, can have severe implications for the mental well-being of the patient, with depression, sleep disturbances, and ultimately suicidal behavior or euthanasia a distinct possibility. In our population, almost two thirds of patients demonstrated a history of and/or a present major mood or anxiety disorder. Two patients committed suicide because they could not endure their constant pain, with another patient having submitted a euthanasia request. This also demonstrates the need for improved psychological/psychiatric screening, and follow-up for these patients. Moreover, although TNP is a relatively rare condition, it still places a significant economic burden on society as 80% of those affected are removed from the workforce, and placed on invalidity benefit.

The GG probably plays the same role in the transmission of pain from the trigeminal branches as the Dorsal Root Ganglia for the rest of the body (cervical, thoracic, lumbar and sacral area). [11, 12] As with the Dorsal Root ganglion, the GG is somatotopically arranged, allowing us to stimulate painful conditions in different areas of the face. Stimulation of the DRG generates excellent results for neuropathic pain, for example in the foot, so we anticipated similar success following stimulation of the GG for neuropathic facial pain. [12] Although our initial results were very promising, we still see a long- term loss of effect. After a positive test stimulation for 77.3% of cases (within the range of 47-80% mentioned by Holsheimer [3], the majority of patients (88%) reported a satisfactory initial pain reduction of at least 50%. However, only 44% of patients still reported satisfactory pain relief at long-term follow-up. Average pain VAS-scores fell from 9/10 to 4/10, 2 weeks after the intervention, then increased again to 7/10 upon last recall. Just over half of the patients (56%) reported a total relapse back to their original pain levels. 13% reported a partial upward creep in pain levels, and only 31% experienced a permanent reduction in pain. With almost all total relapses (80%) occurring between 6 and 24 months after initiation of NS therapy, the incidence of a positive outcome (at least some pain reduction) at 6 months is 93.8%, falling to 46.7% after 24 months of follow-up.

We found a positive predictive value of 44% for a long-term satisfactory effect from NS treatment following a positive test stimulation. This compared to predictive values of 83% and 82% respectively, reported by Holsheimer [3] and Mehrkens and Steude [7], for a greater than 50% reduction in long-term pain. When looking at the underlying reasons for the failure of stimulation therapy long-term, only 50% of cases (5/10) reported failure due to an intrinsic loss of effectiveness of the treatment modality. For the remainder, the treatment failed following an external event (e.g. trauma, tumor relapse), or because of a complication (intra-oral erosion (1), dislocation (1), fibrosis (1)) leading to the patient requesting removal of the stimulator device. Taking into account only those relapses due to an intrinsic failure of the NS therapy, the predictive value of the trial stimulation rose to 80%, which is more in line with previously reported values.

Considering that the majority (82.4%) of these patients suffered from one or more complication, chief among these being fibrosis at the level of the neck (as described), it is not inconceivable that much greater therapeutic success could be achieved in the near future by designing a longer lead, able to tunnel to the infraclavicular region, burying the connector in the infraclavicular fossa pocket, where the IPG is implanted. Initially, we tunneled the lead through a retroauricular track, an area with poor subcutaneous fat, which lead to erosion and development of fibrotic tissue. At present, we directly tunnel the lead to the infraclavicular pocket. The next generation of leads will be designed to connect directly (without an extension lead) to the IPG.

Another adverse event that was observed was the incidence of uncomplicated local infections, which was slightly higher than the 3% reported by Mehrkens and Steude [7], or the incidence seen with SCS. [6, 7] With the technique we developed, using EM neuronavigation technology to guide the needle towards the fora- men ovale, with the lead designed to fit the foramen ovale (tripolar, with close contacts, tined to avoid detachment, and with a bent stylet for good contact with the ganglion), we were able to acquire good therapeutic results, and to reduce the incidence of avoidable complications such as dislocation of the lead.

The small study population (22 subjects) limited the power of the analyses that we could reliably perform. Only a few risk factors could be identified that correlated with a negative outcome. For instance, the presence of anesthesia dolorosa, a well-known pathology influencing the outcome of SCS therapy in a negative manner, could not be identified as a significant risk factor. [6, 13] However, three variables showed a significant correlation with a negative outcome in the long term (e.g. 24 months). These were a young age, no previous peripheral ablative procedure, and no previous peripheral or central pulsed radiofrequency treatment. Younger patients suffered more from physical complications, whereas older patients showed a substantially higher rate of mechanical complications. These findings may reflect the difficulty that older patients had in understanding how to regulate instrument settings. The greatest problems for the younger patient set were tissue responses to the implant. The known negative effects associated with (ab)use issues such as alcohol use have been described previously 10 and were reiterated in this study. These issues occurred mostly with patients who displayed patterns of abusive behavior, and should be considered as a yellow flag for intervention unless these patients can be admitted for withdrawal under psychiatric or psychological follow-up, prior to intervention.

One should take into account that the correlates described only describe a relationship, and are not causal. It is also important to emphasize that this study was established in a retrospective manner with a small patient population, so conclusions derived from our data should be interpreted with caution.

Conclusion

A pharmacological approach, although still the treatment of choice for TNP, often fails to provide satisfactory pain relief, with risks associated with the medications themselves and their usefulness. While the indications for invasive neurodestructive procedures remain unclear, aggravation of pain symptoms occurs for 73% of patients who undergo those procedures. [3, 5, 7-9] This unsatisfactory finding leaves considerable room for improvement, with a need for new treatment options. For patients with persistent TNP, which causes a high level of suffering and associated societal burden, we propose a relatively new method of treatment: a custom-made neurostimulator at the level of the Gasserian ganglion. When tried following a positive test stimulation in 77.3% of the patients, long-term satisfactory pain relief occurred in 44% of these patients after 24 months. Considering only failures due to intrinsic malfunction of the NS therapy (i.e. not technical), the predictive value of the trial stimulation amounted to 80%. This confirms the value of performing a test stimulation to select patients suitable for this treatment modality. The majority (82.4%) of these patients suffered from one or more complications, with neck discomfort due to fibrotic tissue surrounding the connecting piece between the lead and extension being the most frequent complaint (occurring in 50% of patients). These findings are now being used, in collaboration with the lead manufacturer, to improve the design of the electrode, so that we can avoid these complications in the future. Due to the limited size of our study population (22 subjects), we could draw only limited conclusions for criteria leading to a negative outcome. We found that our younger patients were more at risk of physical complications, whereas older patients were less able to operate the NS apparatus, and were more likely to encounter mechanical complications.

Stimulation of the Gasserian ganglion appears to be a promising technique for the treatment of refractory TNP and should be placed in the algorithm of invasive treatment options, a step before either motor cortex stimulation or deep brain stimulation, both of which are more invasive. As a minimally invasive technique, refractory TNP patients should be referred earlier to pain management centers familiar with this technique, as related literature on SCS has indicated the benefits of early treatment. The lessons learnt from this study regarding the pathology of TNP, the specific patient population, and the appropriate lead design and implant techniques, should enable us to improve our ability to treat refractory neuropathic pain in the not too distant future.

References

1. Burchiel KJ. A new classification for facial pain. *Neurosurgery*. 2003;53:1164-1166; discussion 1166-1167.
2. Benoliel R, Eliav E. Neuropathic orofacial pain. *Oral Maxillofac Surg Clin North Am*. 2008;20:237-254, vii.
3. Holsheimer J. Electrical stimulation of the trigeminal tract in chronic, intractable facial neuralgia. *Arch Physiol Biochem*. 2001;109:304-308.
4. Van Buyten JP. Radiofrequency or neuromodulation treatment of chronic pain, when is it useful? . *European Journal of Pain* 2008;Suppl 2:57-66.
5. Sweet WH. Percutaneous methods for the treatment of trigeminal neuralgia and other faciocephalic pain; comparison with microvascular decompression. *Semin Neurol*. 1988;8:272-279.
6. Rizvi S, Kumar K. Spinal cord stimulation for chronic pain: the importance of early referral. *Pain Manag*. 2014;4:329-331.
7. Mehrkens JH, Steude U. Chronic electrostimulation of the trigeminal ganglion in trigeminal neuropathy: current state and future prospects. *Acta Neurochir Suppl*. 2007;97:91-97.
8. Meyerson BA, Hakanson S. Suppression of pain in trigeminal neuropathy by electric stimulation of the gasserian ganglion. *Neurosurgery*. 1986;18:59-66.
9. Van Buyten JP, Linderoth B. Invasive neurostimulation in facial pain and headache syndromes. *European Journal of Pain Supplements*. 2011;5:409-421.
10. Osenbach R. Neurostimulation for the Treatment of Intractable Facial Pain *Pain Medicine*. 2006;7.
11. Al-Kaisy A, Palmisani S, Smith T, Harris S, Pang D. The use of 10-kilohertz spinal cord stimulation in a cohort of patients with chronic neuropathic limb pain refractory to medical management. *Neuromodulation*. 2015;18:18-23; discussion 23.
12. Van Buyten JP, Smet I, Liem L, Russo M, Huygen F. Stimulation of dorsal root ganglia for the management of complex regional pain syndrome: a prospective case series. *Pain Pract*. 2015;15:208-216.
13. Sindou MP, Mertens P, Bendavid U, Garcia-Larrea L, Mauguiere F. Predictive value of somatosensory evoked potentials for long-lasting pain relief after spinal cord stimulation: practical use for patient selection. *Neurosurgery*. 2003;52:1374-1383; discussion 1383-1374.

We used electromagnetic neuronavigation to improve precision of the electrode placement.

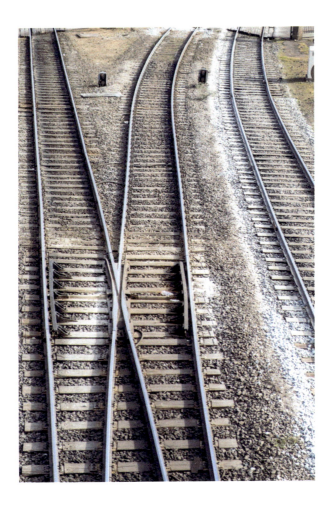

Chapter 4
Electromagnetic Navigation Technology for More Precise Electrode Placement in the Foramen Ovale: A Technical Report

Jean-Pierre Van Buyten[1], Iris Smet[1], Erik Van de Kelft[2]

1 Department of Anesthesia and Pain Management, AZ Nikolaas, Sint-Niklaas, Belgium
2 Department of Neurosurgery, AZ Nikolaas, Sint-Niklaas, Belgium

Neuromodulation: technology at the neural interface:2009: 12 (3): 244-249

Abstract

Introduction

Interventional pain management techniques require precise positioning of needles or electrodes, therefore fluoroscopic control is mandatory. This imaging technique does however not visualize soft tissues such as blood vessels. Moreover, patient and physician are exposed to a considerable dose of radiation. Computed tomography (CT)-scans give a better view of soft tissues, but there use requires presence of a radiologist and has proven to be laborious and time consuming.

Objectives

This study is to develop a technique using electromagnetic (EM) navigation as a guidance technique for interventional pain management, using CT and/or magnetic resonance (MRI) images uploaded on the navigation station.

Methods

One of the best documented interventional procedures for the management of trigeminal neuralgia is percutaneous radiofrequency treatment of the Gasserian ganglion. EM navigation software for intracranial applications already exists. We developed a technique using a stylet with two magnetic coils suitable for EM navigation. The procedure is followed in real time on a computer screen where the patient's multislice CT-scan images and three-dimensional reconstruction of his face are uploaded. Virtual landmarks on the screen are matched with those on the patient's face, calculating the precision of the needle placement.

Discussion

The experience with EM navigation acquired with the radiofrequency technique can be transferred to other interventional pain management techniques, for instance, for the placement of a neuromodulation electrode close to the Gasserian ganglion. Currently, research is ongoing to extend the software of the navigation station for spinal application, and to adapt neurostimulation hardware to the EM navigation technology. This technology will allow neuromodulation techniques to be performed without x-ray exposure for the patient and the physician, and this with the precision of CT/MR imaging guidance.

Key words
Chronic pain, electromagnetic neuronavigation, electrode placement, radiofrequency, trigeminal neuralgia.

Introduction

Trigeminal neuralgia (TN) also referred to as "tic douloureux" is an extremely painful condition. When pharmacologic treatment fails to provide satisfactory pain relief or causes intolerable side-effects, interventional pain management techniques may be indicated. Several interventional treatment possibilities exist such as glycerol injection into the Gasserian Ganglion, radiofrequency (RF) thermo lesion of the Gasserian Ganglion, balloon compression into the ganglion, and micro vascular decompression surgery (Janetta operation). The selection of the interventional technique is mainly guided by the patient's age and general condition. [1-3] Certainly, for older patients with frequent co-morbidity, the minimal invasive percutaneous techniques are preferred. [1,4] RF treatment of the Gasserian ganglion for the management of TN is probably the oldest documented radiofrequency procedure [5]; although no randomized controlled trials are published, the efficacy was documented in large patient series. [6] Radiofrequency thermo lesioning of the Gasserian ganglion can induce neurologic complications such dysesthesia, anesthesia dolorosa, and diminished corneal reflex (6). More recently pulsed radiofrequency (PRF) also is used. This is an adapted RF technique whereby the high frequency current is delivered in bursts of 20 msec followed by a silent period of 480 msec allowing the generated heat to be washed and thereby taking care that the temperature at the electrode tip does not exceed 42°C, thus reducing the risk for neurologic complications. [7] Patients suffering TN who cannot adequately be controlled by pharmacologic treatment receive extensive explanation on the potential interventional treatment options. Based on the patient's general condition, a microvascular decompression surgery or a radiofrequency treatment is proposed. The patient helps selecting between treatment options after having received information relative to expected duration of action and potential complications of the treatment.

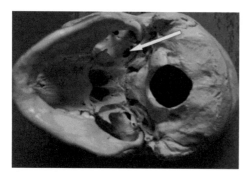

Figure 1: The arrow shows the left foramen ovale.

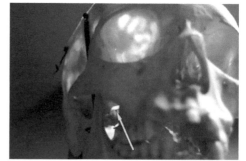

Figure 2: The arrow indicates the track of the needle.

The success rate of these interventions depends largely on the precision with which the Gasserian Ganglion is reached. We introduced the use of electromagnetic (EM) navigation technology to improve precision of the electrode placement. The use of this navigation technique has been reported in cardiology [8], but to our knowledge its application for the correct electrode insertion in the foramen ovale was not described yet.

The experience gathered with the RF electrode placement with EM navigation will help to expand its use to other pain management techniques such as neuromodulation procedures.

Radiofrequency treatment of the Gasserian Ganglion

The Gasserian ganglion is commonly reached through the foramen ovale. (Figure 1). The needle trajectory is indicated in Figure 2. Correct identification of the foramen ovale and progressive insertion of the electrode requires different fluoroscopic controls. For patient's comfort the procedure is performed under mild sedation. The patient must be awakened to be able to report sensation upon sensory stimulation at 50 Hz. When electro-stimulation confirms the fluoroscopically observed correct needle placement, the patient is again sedated to perform the thermo lesion or PRF treatment. The use of imaging technique exposes the patient and the physician to high dose radiation. Because of the danger of long-term x-ray exposure, it is impossible to do real time follow-up of the needle trajectory. The fluoroscopy has the disadvantage to give you only a two-dimensional view of the procedure. Moreover, with conventional x-rays it is not always easy to view the foramen ovale and soft tissues such as blood vessels are not visualized. Therefore, occasional puncturing of the facial artery leading to postoperative hematoma occurs.

Alternatively, computed tomography (CT)-scan guided techniques have been proposed. 9. This imaging technique allows visualization of the soft tissue and is consequently more accurate. This allows you real time follow-up and the trajectory of the needle is followed in three dimensions with a coronal, axial, and sagittal view. An example of a CT-scan with insertion of the needle in the foramen ovale is given in Figure 3. We used this technique for several years but the obligatory presence of a radiologist, and the longer time needed to perform the procedure both contribute the patient's discomfort and a higher cost for the hospital. In our department, more than 90 procedures treating TN have been carried out with the CT-guided technique, yielding good results with great precision and without any technical or medical complication.

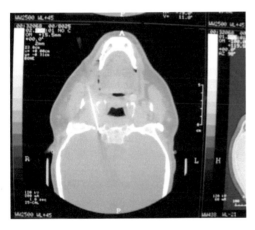
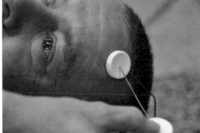

Figure 3: Computed tomography-guided placement of the needle through the foramen ovale.

Figure 4: Noninvasive dynamic reference frame.

EM Navigation Guided Procedure

The introduction of navigation technology in surgery triggered the idea of using this technology for interventional management techniques. Classical navigation with infrared camera proved to be time consuming and not very accurate. EM tracking, however, allows navigating with needles under "real time" supervision. Needles suitable for EM navigation, and allowing real time monitoring of the needle placement during percutaneous pain management techniques, have been developed (AZ Nikolaas, Sint- Nikolaas, Belgium in cooperation with the Surgical Navigation Technology, a company based in

Denver (Col) USA, presently known as Medtronic-SNT). Because there is a technical note there is no need for ethical committee approval. The navigation needle is in fact a stylet equipped with two magnetic coils, inserted into the thermo couple needle, normally used for the RF procedure.

First a multislice CT-scan is taken of the area between the puncture (entry point) of the skin and the target (the foramen ovale). The best scans where the target is most visible in coronal, axial and sagittal view are downloaded from the hospital network or from an optical disc to the computer of the navigation system.

During the procedures, the patient's head is positioned upon a magnet and so maintained within a magnetic field.

Certain reference points on the three-dimensional reconstruction of the face are ticked into the computer by simple mouse click. The same reference points are indicated with a coiled stylet applied to the face and sent to the navigation machine by pushing a foot switch. One reference point (antenna) is fixed to the frontal area of the skull. (Figure 4)

This point also is entered into the computer, thus situating the position of the patient within the magnetic field, and allowing the patient to move without causing any loss of precision of the representation. The track is dotted out virtually on the computer screen. (Figure 5)

The computer, matching virtual landmarks on the three- dimensional reconstruction of the face with the same land- marks on the patient's face, then calculates the circle with a precision of approximately 1 mm within which we can work. The coiled stylet is introduced into the thermocouple needle and then we can navigate real time following exactly the virtual track toward the foramen ovale (Figure 6). Once our needle passes the foramen a short control of the position of the needle is made by a one shot fluoroscopic image not lasting longer than 1 sec. By removing the coiled stylet, we lose contact with the magnetic field and the navigation station.

Because of the real-time visualization of the needle placement (Figure 7) the procedure can be performed under local anesthesia or light propofol sedation. Considering that patients treated by RF of the Gasserian ganglion are mainly elderly and frail, sedation increases patient's comfort and safety of the intervention.

Discussion

The percutaneous approach of the foramen ovale is sometimes difficult because of the unclear visualization of the foramen with fluoroscopy and the many anatomic variations of this foramen. This fact leads to long x-ray exposure of medical staff and patients and jeopardizes the success of an otherwise very successful procedure. EM navigation makes this procedure simpler, safer, more accurate, faster, and less invasive.

Electromagnetic Neuronavigation

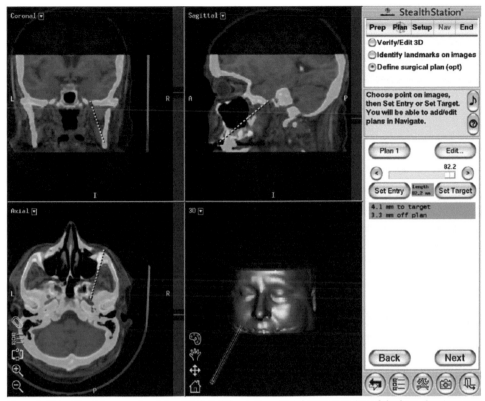

Figure 5: Virtual track in coronal, axial, sagittal, and three-dimensional reconstruction of the face, showing entry and target point.

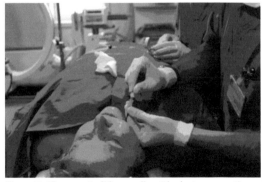

Figure 6: Placement of the needle with electromagnetic navigation guidance.

Chapter 4

Our pain center works closely together with the department of neurosurgery to perform these procedures. Since the first introduction several procedures have been carried out. After a short learning period, we are now able to do three procedures within one hour because most of the programming work can be performed outside the operating room. EM navigation use in interventional pain therapy was, to our knowledge, not reported earlier. In the near future, this technology will be used for other applications within interventional pain management and neurosurgery. CT images are by far more precise than the classical fluoroscopy images. The exposure to x-rays of the physician is much higher using CT guidance as compared with fluoroscopy. The use of EM navigation bypasses this step for the physician and allows working with CT precision and without x-ray exposure. Software for spine surgery is yet available. If the industry can adapt neurostimulation hard- ware to EM navigation technology by, for example, developing coiled stylets to introduce into the spinal cord stimulation leads, we will be able to do CT-guided, real time imaging for spinal cord stimulation, thus decreasing considerably the exposure time to x-rays, and increasing the comfort of the medical staff by making radioprotection during the procedures useless. Once the technology of following flexible instruments like leads is developed, we are only one step away from using this technology in many other applications where leads and catheters have to be followed or guided.

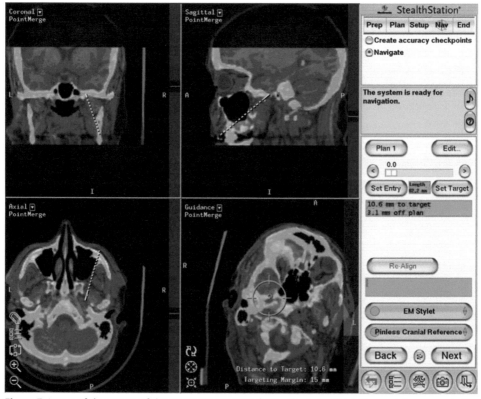

Figure 7: Image of the screen of the navigation station during the procedure. Green dot represents the tip of the needle.

References

1. Aphelbaum R. Advantages and disadvantages of various techniques to treat trigeminal neuralgia. In: Rovit R, Murali R, Janetta P, eds. *Trigeminal Neuralgia*. Baltimore MD: Wiliams & Wilkins; 1990. 239-250.
2. Zakrzewska JM, Thomas DG. Patient's assessment of outcome after three surgical procedures for the management of trigeminal neuralgia. *Acta Neurochir (Wien)*. 1993;122:225-230.
3. Lopez BC, Hamlyn PJ, Zakrzewska JM. Systematic review of ablative neurosurgical techniques for the treatment of trigeminal neuralgia. *Neurosurgery*. 2004;54:973-982; discussion 982-973.
4. Janetta P. Trigeminal Neuralgia: Treatment by microvascular decompression. In: Wilkins R, Regachary S, eds. *Neurosurgery*. New York: McGrawy-Hill; 1996. 3961-3968.
5. Sweet WH, Wepsic JG. Controlled thermocoagulation of trigeminal ganglion and root for differential destruction of pain fibers. Part I : Trigeminal neuralgia. *J Neurosurg*. 1974;39:143-156.
6. Kanpolat Y, Savas A, Bekar A, Berk C. Percutaneous controlled radiofrequency trigeminal rhizotomy for the treatment of idiopathic trigeminal neuralgia: 25-year experience with 1,600 patients. *Neurosurgery*. 2001;48:524-532; discussion 532-524.
7. Van Zundert J, Brabant S, Van de Kelft E, Vercruyssen A, Van Buyten JP. Pulsed radiofrequency treatment of the Gasserian ganglion in patients with idiopathic trigeminal neuralgia. *Pain*. 2003;104:449-452.
8. Saoudi N, Ricard P, Yaici K. Magnetic navigation and voltage mapping guided implantation of a pacemaker atrial lead in a previously unpaceable patient. *Europace*. 2007;9:1194-1195.
9. Kanpolat Y, Savas A, Bekar A, Berk C. CT-guided pain procedures. *Neurochirurgie*. 1990;36:394-398.

We used phenotyping to define subgroups of patients with medically refractory headache that are more likely to respond to occipital nerve stimulation, which is an indirect stimulation via the trigeminocervical complex.

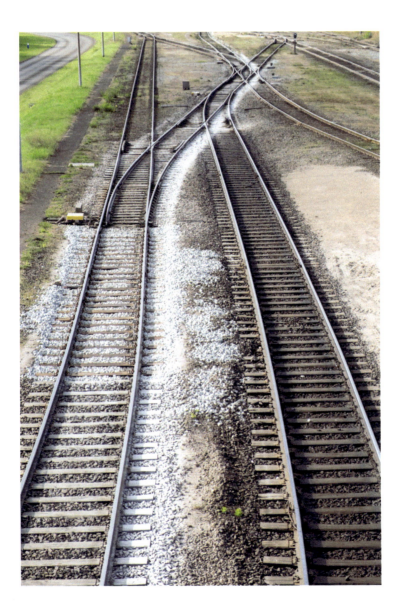

Chapter 5
Phenotype of patients responsive to occipital nerve stimulation for refractory head pain

K Paemeleire[1], J-P Van Buyten[2], M Van Buynder[3], D Alicino[3], G Van Maele[3], I Smet[2] and PJ Goadsby[4]

1 Department of Neurology, Ghent, Belgium.
2 Pain Clinic, AZ Nikolaas, Sint-Niklaas, Belgium.
3 Medical Informatics & Statistics, Ghent University Hospital, Ghent, Belgium.
4 Headache Group, Department of Neurology, University of California, San Francisco, San Francisco, CA, USA.

*K.P and J-P.V.B. contributed equally to this publication.

Abstract

Occipital nerve stimulation (ONS) has been employed off-label for medically refractory head pain. Identification of specific headache diagnoses responding to this modality of treatment is required. Forty-four patients with medically refractory head pain and treated with ONS were invited to participate in a retrospective study including a clinical interview and, if necessary, an indomethacin test to establish the headache phenotype according to the International Classification of Headache Disorders, 2nd ed (ICHD-II). We gathered data from questionnaires before implantation, at 1 month after implantation, and at long-term follow-up. Twenty-six patients consented and were phenotyped. At 1 month follow-up and at long-term follow-up a significant decrease in all pain parameters was noted, as well as in analgesic use. Quality of sleep and quality of life improved. Patient satisfaction was generally high as 80% of patients had ≥ 50% pain relief at long-term follow-up. The overall complication rate was low, but revisions were frequent. After phenotyping, two main groups emerged: eight patients had 'Migraine without aura' (ICHD-II 1.1) and eight patients 'Constant pain caused by compression, irritation or distortion of cranial nerves or upper cervical roots by structural lesions' (ICHD-II 13.12). Overuse of symptomatic acute headache treatments was associated with less favorable long-term outcome in migraine patients. We conclude that careful clinical phenotyping may help in defining subgroups of patients with medically refractory headache that are more likely to respond to ONS. The data suggest medication overuse should be managed appropriately when considering ONS in migraine. A controlled prospective study for ONS in ICHD-II 13.12 is warranted.

Keywords
Occipital neurostimulation, refractory headache, neuropathic pain, migraine

Introduction

Headache is among the most common reasons for patients to seek medical care. Migraine, the most common form of disabling primary headache, has been estimated to be the most common form of disabling primary headache, has been estimated to be the most costly neurological disorder in the European Community[1] Although considerable developments have been made in understanding and treating primary headache, there remains a group of patients with difficult to treat headache problems, labelled generically as medically intractable headache.[2]. In general terms these patients have frequent, daily or near-daily headache unresponsive to medical therapy. Neuromodulation methods may offer an opportunity to address the needs of these highly-disabled patients. In a landmark paper, Weiner and Reed described excellent outcomes with occipital neurostimulation (ONS) in 12 patients described as having occipital neuralgia.[3] On clinical review of this patient cohort and using the International Classification of Headache Disorders, 2nd ed (ICHD-II)4, it became clear that most of them had chronic migraine and one had hemicrania continua. A subsequent positron emission tomography study in those with chronic migraine [5] demonstrated persistent activation of the dorsolateral pons, as is seen in other imaging studies of migraine [6], and activation of thalamus structures when the device was activated.

Given that there has been off-label use of ONS on compassionate grounds in highly disabled patients, there is an opportunity to classify those patients using the ICHD-II in order to identify potential patient groups for systematic study. Recent experience with chronic cluster headache suggests that ONS may be of help in that disorder.[7, 8] Indeed, other modalities of stimulation have begun to be used in chronic cluster headache, specifically deep brain stimulation, and these are also proving highly promising.[9] Data from the first randomized, controlled, prospective trial for ONS for the Treatment of Intractable Migraine headache (ONSTIM trial) have recently become available in abstract form.[10] The results indicate that ONS may be a promising treatment for some intractable chronic migraine patients, and further controlled trials are required. Interestingly, given the hemicrania continua patient in Weiner and Reed's initial cohort3, there are nine cases of hemicrania continua treated with ONS now reported in the literature, and seven benefited from the therapy. [11-13] These cases are important, since hemicrania continua is an indomethacin-sensitive headache, which broadens still the range of headache types that may benefit from this approach. Results of ONS in primary headache disorders have recently been reviewed.[14]

In this retrospective study a cohort of patients, implanted with occipital neurostimulators at a single site, were invited to attend clinical evaluation and, if necessary, to undergo an indomethacin test in order to clarify the diagnosis. We confirm other reports that chronic migraine patients can be treated with this approach, adding a note of caution around medication overuse, and identify a previously unreported group, Upper Cervical Neuropathic Pain (ICHD-II, 13.12), who have a promising outcome. This work was presented in preliminary form at the 10th Congress of the European Federation of Neurological Societies (Brussels, August 2008 [15]).

Methods

Forty-four patients had been consecutively treated with ONS for medically refractory headache between April 2000 and December 2006 at the AZ Nikolaas Pain Clinic (J-P.V.B, Figure 1). ONS therapy was offered to these patients as part of the regular pain program, and the decision to offer this treatment to the patient was made by the pain physician based on a working diagnosis of occipital neuralgia or cervicogenic headache, and after all patients had undergone a preoperative psychological evaluation. The Ethics Committees of the Ghent University Hospital in Ghent and the AZ Nikolaas in Sint-Niklaas approved the study (EC/2006/383). Informed consent was sought from all patients by letter to review their clinical data, including a pre-implantation questionnaire, a questionnaire at 1 month following trial stimulation (i.e. before the definitive implantation procedure), as well as technical details: implantation date and procedure; complications such as dislocations, lead fractures, electrical leakage at the connections and infection; and battery replacement. The patients were invited by letter to be interviewed by an independent and blinded headache neurologist at the Department of Neurology of the Ghent University Hospital (K.P.). If necessary to make a specific headache diagnosis, patients were invited to give their informed consent to undergo an indomethacin test, either intra- muscular or oral. The indomethacin tests were per- formed by the treating physician at AZ Nikolaas Pain Clinic (J-P.V.B.). Patients who entered the study were finally invited to fill out the post-implantation questionnaire for a second time at their last visit at AZ Nikolaas Pain Clinic, to obtain long-term follow-up data.

Implantation technique

Initially, the implantation technique described by Weiner and Reed 3 was used. A subcutaneous lead was inserted towards the midline via a lateral incision close to the mastoid process. The procedure was done under propofol sedation with a wake up during the procedure in order to check the area of paresthesia. With growing experience the technique was adapted and the ONS procedure is now performed under general anesthesia with the patient in the prone position and the head in a horseshoe headrest. The incision was made close to the occiput, where there is more fat tissue that affords a subcutaneous pocket substantial enough for adequate fixation of the lead and leaving a loop. A curved needle (custom made by Medtronic Inc., Bakken Research Centre, Maastricht, the Netherlands) was pushed from the occiput towards the mastoid process in the subcutaneous tissue, to cross the greater, lesser and least occipital nerve. The position of the lead was checked with fluoroscopy after the needle had been pulled out. An intermediate incision was made in the suprascapular area, again creating a pocket, and a second loop was left behind. A third incision was made parallel to the spine at the high thoracic level to bury the connection between the lead and the temporary extension lead. The connection was fixated to the underlying tissue. The temporary extension lead was tunneled laterally over the thoracic wall. After a successful trial period of at least 1 month, a pocket was created in the gluteal area for the implantable pulse generator, a new extension lead was tunneled towards the connector and the new connector was secured to the underlying tissue. Stimulation parameters, including frequency, pulse width and voltage, were adjusted so that all patients experienced mild paresthesia in the stimulated area.

Pain questionnaires

The pre- and post-implantation questionnaires were developed in 1997 by the Belgian Pain Society (the Belgian Chapter of the International Association for the Study of Pain). Pain data are gathered with a visual analogue scale (VAS), but the questionnaire has otherwise not been validated. These evaluation forms are required by the Belgian government for reimbursement of all patients with chronic pain treated with implantable devices (neurostimulators and intrathecal drug-delivery pumps). The questionnaires include data on regional distribution of the pain using a pre-printed drawing of the head and body, pain severity scores on a VAS from 0 to 10 indicating 'pain at present', 'worst pain last week', 'lowest pain last week', 'average pain last week', percentage pain-free time (0–100%), average daily number of analgesics used, quality of sleep on a scale from 1 to 5, influence of pain on activities of daily living, social activities, independence of others, hobbies and need for bed rest (all the five using VAS scores on a scale from 0 to 10). The post-implantation questionnaire was filled out by every patient after 1 month of stimulation and by 21 patients at long-term follow-up. This questionnaire included data on the subjective area of stimulation on a pre-printed drawing, perceived pain relief ('worse', 'too little', 'moderate', 'largely', 'almost complete', 'complete'), patient satisfaction ('excellent', 'very good', 'good', 'moderate', 'poor', 'no effect' or 'worse'), and the question whether the patient would undergo the procedure again for the same indication, but was otherwise identical to the pre-implantation questionnaire.

Clinical interview

During the clinical interview demographic data, analgesic use, all necessary information to make a headache diagnosis according to ICHD-II 4, as well as percent- age of pain relief at long-term follow-up, were recorded. To make a diagnosis of medication overuse headache the Appendix Criteria were used.[16] Patients were instructed not to discuss their pre-implantation diagnosis. All clinical data were made available to a second blinded headache neurologist (P.J.G.) before clinical diagnoses were assigned.

Indomethacin testing

To exclude a diagnosis of paroxysmal hemicrania or hemicrania continua an intramuscular indomethacin test was performed in some patients with strictly uni- lateral (attacks of) head pain.[17] Intramuscular indomethacin tests were performed at the Pain Clinic of AZ Nikolaas. Patients had their stimulator turned off in the morning and recorded pain on a VAS from 0 to 10 for 3 h in a diary. If the head pain reached an intensity of ≥ 5/10 on the VAS, 100 mg indomethacin was injected intramuscularly. Pain scores were recorded each hour afterwards for the rest of the day. Afterwards the patients received instructions to switch the stimulator back on. If the head pain reached an intensity of < 5/10 during the 3-h observation period, instructions were given to perform an ambulatory oral indomethacin test. Patients would record headache intensity on an hourly basis in a headache diary while under indomethacin. Indomethacin was started at 25 mg three times per day for 3 days. If the patient was not pain free, the indomethacin dose was increased to 50 mg three times per day for 3 days. If the patient was not pain free, the indomethacin dose was further increased to 75 mg three times per day for 3 days. If the patient was not completely pain free at that point in time, the oral indomethacin test was deemed negative. Exclusion criteria for an indomethacin test were asthma, renal disease, allergy to acetylsalicylic acid or non-steroidal anti-inflammatory drugs, active peptic ulcer disease and pregnancy.

Data analysis

Statistical analysis of the data was performed by an independent statistician (G.V.M.) with R, a language and environment for statistical computing.[18] Univariate comparison of unpaired groups was done with Fisher's exact test for categorical data and the non-parametric Mann–Whitney U-test for the comparison of continuous variables. The non-parametric Friedman two-way ANOVA test with Wilcoxon matched-pairs signed-ranks test as multiple range test was used to compare measurements over the three time intervals. The significance level was set at a ¼ 0.05, two-tailed.

Results

All 44 patients consented to have their data used from the questionnaires pre-implantation and at 1 month post-implantation. Twenty-six patients consented to undergo clinical interview, which took place at the Neurology Department of the Ghent University Hospital between December 2006 and April 2007. Data from the questionnaire at long-term follow-up were additionally obtained from 21 of these 26 patients. One patient's records (including all three questionnaires) could not be retrieved, but the patient (no. 6) presented for the clinical interview.

Overall safety in all 44 patients

The mean age of all 44 patients at implantation was 48 years (range 29–75). All 44 patients had an occipital component to their head pain and 18 also had a trigeminal component. Twenty-one patients underwent unilateral neurostimulation, 10 on the left, 11 on the right, and 23 had bilateral neurostimulation, using one electrode in 19 and two electrodes in four.

The mean duration of follow-up was 36 months (range 7–87 months). The total device time was 1592 months. Fourteen of the 44 patients had a total of 18 revisions. Eleven patients had to have a new lead put in place, in two patients because of dislocation, using the initial technique with a lateral incision (cf. Methods section), and in the other nine patients because of lead fracture, with four of these patients undergoing a second revision, again lead replacement. In three cases, there was a problem with the connection, with pain due to local current leakage, requiring opening of the connection and cleaning it. There were two instances of infection, one at the level of the lead insert during the trial period, and one later after implantation at the level of the connector due to a small skin defect. Both infections were resolved with short-term antibiotic treatment.

Pooled results for the 26 phenotyped patients

Twenty-six of the 44 patients (59%) agreed to be phenotyped. Pooled outcome data for this group are summarized in Table 1. Statistically significant improvements were obtained on all outcome

Chapter 5

Table 1. Pooled results for the twenty-six phenotyped patients

Parameter	Pre-implantation	At 1 month's follow-up	At long-term follow-up
1. Pain VAS scores	Mean (range) VAS score	Mean (range) VAS score	Mean (range) VAS score
Pain at present	7.3 (2.5–10)	2.6 (1–6)*	2.6 (1–7)†
Worst pain last week	8.9 (5.5–10)	4.8 (1–10)*	5.7 (1–9)†
Lowest pain last week	5.3 (1–10)	1.8 (1–4)*	2.5 (1–6)†‡
Average pain last week	7.3 (3.5–10)	2.6 (1–5.5)*	3.9 (1–7)†‡
2. Long-term pain relief		Mean percentage (range)	Mean percentage (range)
		72.2% (0–100%)*	63% (0–100%)
3. Time spent pain free	Mean percentage (range)	Mean percentage (range)	Mean percentage (range)
	7.3% (0–40%)	72.2% (0–100%)*	56.7% (0–100%)†‡
4. Analgesic consumption	Mean number (range) of analgesics/day	Mean number (range) of analgesics/day	Mean number (range) of analgesics/day
	2.9 (1–4)	1.5 (0–4)*	1.6 (0–4)†
5. Quality of life	Mean (range) VAS score	Mean (range) VAS score	Mean (range) VAS score
Influence of pain on activities of daily living	6.3 (2–9)	3.6 (1–8)*	3.6 (1–9)†
Influence of pain on social activities	7.4 (2–10)	3.2 (1–8)*	3.8 (1–9)†
Influence of pain on independence of others	3.7 (1–10)	1.9 (1–5)*	2.1 (1–9)†
Influence of pain on hobbies	7.4 (1–10)	3.9 (1–9.5)*	4 (1–9)†
Influence of pain on need for bedrest	5.8 (1–10)	2.7 (1–8.5)*	2.7 (1–5)†
6. Quality of sleep	Mean percentage scoring sleep at least good	Mean percentage scoring sleep at least good	Mean percentage scoring sleep at least good
	56%	83%*	86%†

*Significant change (P < 0.05) in parameter at 1 month's follow-up compared with pre-implantation status.
†Significant change (P < 0.05) in parameter at long-term follow-up compared with pre-implantation status.
‡Significant change (P < 0.05) in parameter at long-term follow-up compared with 1 month's follow-up status.

parameters, both at 1 month's follow-up and at long-term follow-up when compared with pre-implantation data. The mean percentage long-term pain relief was 63% (range 0– 100%), and 81% (21 of 26) of the patients had at least 50% long-term pain relief. The outcome on three parameters was significantly worse at long-term follow-up compared with data at 1 month post implantation, including increased 'lowest pain last week', increased 'average pain last week' and decreased percentage time spent pain free.

Data from questionnaires on all available para- meters were compared between patients who volunteered for a clinical interview (n = 26) and those who did not (n = 18) at baseline and at 1 month's follow-up. There were no significant differences except for the included patients being older (average of 51 vs. 44 years old), having less influence of pain on activities of daily living and hobbies at baseline, and having less influence of pain on hobbies at 1 month's follow-up.

Clinical phenotyping

The mean age of the 26 patients who were phenotyped was 51 years at the time of implantation (range 29–75). There were 14 women and 12 men in this group. An indomethacin test was proposed to six patients, of whom two refused. All four indomethacin tests, of which two were oral and two intramuscular, were negative. The clinical diagnoses for all 26 patients fell into nine ICHD-II categories (Fig. 1). Two main subgroups were identified: eight patients with migraine without aura (ICHD-II 1.1) and eight patients with 'Constant pain caused by compression, irritation or distortion of cranial nerves or upper cervical roots by structural lesions' (ICHD-II 13.12). All patients with migraine without aura had an additional diagnosis of medication overuse headache prior to implantation. All migraine patients failed at least four classes of preventive medicines, of which at least three were a b-blocker, anticonvulsant, calcium channel blocker or tricyclic antidepressant, thus fulfilling current criteria for medical intractability.2. We compared all available data between the two groups ICHD-II 1.1 and ICHD-II 13.12 and found that there were few significant differences, except that patients with ICHD-II 13.12 had significantly more pain relief (mean 80% vs. 47%; n = 8 in both groups) at long-term follow-up, and that migraine patients were more independent of others at 1 month's follow-up (n = 8 in both groups). The latter difference was not seen at long-term follow-up.

Patients with migraine

The eight migraine patients had a mean follow-up of 24 months following implantation (range 12–60 months). Patient satisfaction at 1 month's follow-up was rated excellent by one, very good by two and good by five. At long-term follow-up one patient indicated no effect, one only moderate effect, one a good effect, three very good and one excellent (missing data in one patient). At 1 month's follow-up, every patient would undergo a repeat of the procedure, but at long-term follow-up two out of seven patients would not (missing data in one patient). Grouped data from the questionnaires at 1 month and long-term follow-up were compared with the data pre-implantation. There was a significant reduction on most pain parameters ('actual pain', P = 0.00557; 'least pain last week', P = 0.0118; 'mean pain last week', P = 0.00952; '% pain free', P = 0.00298) except for the 'worst pain in the last week' (P = 0.0539). The absolute average value for 'mean pain last week' decreased from 7/10 VAS score pre-implantation to 2.4/10 and 4/10 at 1 month and long-term follow-up,

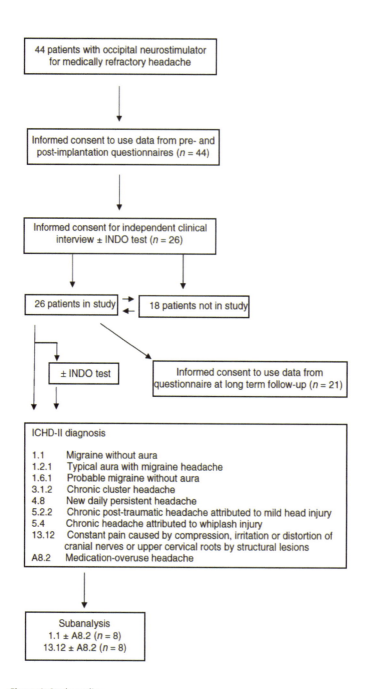

Figure 1: Study outline.

respectively. Five out of seven patients (missing data in one) had at least a three-point drop in 'mean pain last week' at long-term follow-up. The use of analgesics was significantly diminished (P = 0.0469). Influence of pain on most activity para- meters was not significantly changed, except for an increase in social activities (P = 0.0262). Quality of sleep was not significantly changed. There were no significant differences between the data at 1 month's follow-up vs. long-term follow-up, except for a decrease in percentage of time spent pain free at long-term follow-up, which decreased from 71 to 51% (P = 0.04983).

We considered migraine without aura patients with respect to presence (n = 5) or absence (n = 3) of medication overuse headache (see Table 2) at long-term follow-up. The average percentage pain relief at long-term follow-up was 47% for the entire group of eight patients (range 0–95%). Despite the small numbers, patients with medication overuse had significantly less percentage pain relief at long-term follow-up when compared with those without (mean of 28% vs. 78%; P = 0.0498).

Head pain of cervical origin

The eight patients suffering from 'Constant pain caused by compression, irritation or distortion of cranial nerves or upper cervical roots by structural lesions' had a mean follow-up of 53 months following implantation (range 32–74 months). All but one patient had suffered for at least 5 years from 'Constant pain caused by compression, irritation or distortion of cranial nerves or upper cervical roots by structural lesions' despite conventional treatments, which illustrates the intractable nature of their condition (2). Patients (missing data for one patient) rated the procedure as excel- lent (n = 2), very good (n = 2), or at least good (n = 3) at 1 month post implantation. At long-term follow-up (missing data for one patient) satisfaction with the technique was at least good (n = 4), but also very good (n = 1) and excellent (n = 2). All patients indicated they would redo the procedure at 1 month and at long-term follow-up (with data missing for one patient). From our retrospective interview, we ascertained that two of eight patients had maximal pain relief within 24 h after implantation, five of eight patients had an average of 70% (range 40–100%) pain relief within the first 24 h, and all eight patients had an average pain relief of 70% (range 20–100%) within 7 days. Most patients within this group (n = 5) found that switching the stimulator off led to exacerbation of the pain very quickly, within 10 min to 1 h. Delay of pain relief upon switching the stimulator back on varied between 10 min and days. However, two patients were able to switch the stimulator off part of the day to save on battery, but switch it on when the pain exacerbated. Grouped data from the questionnaires at 1 month and long-term follow-up were compared with the data pre-implantation. There was a significant reduction in all pain parameters: 'actual pain' (P = 0.0211), 'worst pain in the last week' (P = 0.00841), 'least pain last week' (P = 0.0160) and 'mean pain last week' (P = 0.0135); the '% pain-free' increased from an average pre-implantation value of 13% to 68% and 53% at 1 month and long-term follow-up, respectively (P = 0.0193). The absolute average value for 'mean pain last week' decreased from 7.4/10 VAS score pre-implantation to 2.9/10 and 4.4/10 at 1 month and long-term follow-up, respectively. Six out of seven patients (missing data in one) had at least a three-point drop in 'mean pain last week' at long-term follow-up. The use of analgesics was significantly diminished (P = 0.0244) and quality of sleep improved (P = 0.0468). Influence of pain on most activity parameters was significantly diminished, specifically activities of daily living (P = 0.0331), social activities (P = 0.0295), dependency on others (P = 0.0246) and need for bed rest (P = 0.0220), except for hobbies (P = 0.0941). There were no significant differences between the data at 1 month's follow-up vs. at long-

Chapter 5

Table 2. Details of migraine patient outcomes

Patient	Baseline ICHD-II diagnosis†	VAS scores for pain pre-implantation actual/worst/least/mean				VAS scores for pain at 1 month actual/worst/least/mean				VAS scores for pain long-term actual/worst/least/mean				% pain relief long-term	MO long-term	Redo long-term
1	1.1, A8.2	8.5	9.5	7.5	7.5	1	8	1	2	3	8	2	3	0	Yes	No
5	1.1, A8.2	3.5	7	2.5	3.5	2	3	1	2	MD	7	3	6	0	Yes	No
12	1.1, A8.2	4	10	2	6.5	2	9	—	3	1	5	1	2	80	No	Yes
14	1.1, A8.2	9	10	5	8	1	1	—	1	1	8	1	1	95	No	Yes
16	1.1, A8.2	8	8	2	5	3	5	1	2	2.5	6.5	2	5	60	No	Yes
17	1.1, A8.2	9	10	6.5	9.5	4	10	1	4	MD	MD	MD	MD	30	Yes	MD
24	1.1, A8.2	7	7	7	7	4.5	9	4	4	4.5	9	3	6	60	Yes	Yes
26	1.1, A8.2	9	9	6	9	1	2	1	1	1	5	5	5	50	Yes	Yes

ICHD-II 1.1, 8.2	Number of patients	% pain relief long-term
MO+	5	28%*
MO–	3	78%*

*$P = 0.0498$.
†1.1: Migraine without aura; A8.2: medication overuse headache.
MD, missing data; MO+/–, with or without medication overuse at long-term follow-up.

Table 3. Details of outcome of patients suffering from ICHD-II 13.12—Upper Cervical Neuropathic Pain

Patient	Baseline ICHD-II diagnosis[†]	VAS scores for pain pre-implantation actual/worst/least/mean				VAS scores for pain at 1 month actual/worst/least/mean				VAS scores for pain long-term actual/worst/least/mean				% pain relief long-term	MO long-term	Redo long-term
2	13.12	2.5	10	1	1.5	6	9	1	4.5	1	6	1	3	95	Yes	Yes
3	13.12	8	9	7	8	1	1	–	–	4	9	3	6	75	Yes	Yes
7	13.12	10	10	10	10	4	7	4	4	7	9	6	7	80	No	Yes
8	13.12	7	7.5	4	6.5	4	4	4	3	5.5	5.5	5.5	5.5	100	No	Yes
9	13.12	7.5	9	4	6	1.5	2.5	1	–	1	1	1	–	100	No	Yes
13	13.12	7	10	6	8	4.5	4.5	2	3	3	6	3	4.5	72.5	Yes	Yes
19	13.12	9.5	9.5	9.5	9.5	3	3	3	3	MD	MD	MD	MD	65	Yes	MD
23	13.12	5	9	4	8	3	5.5	2.5	4	3.5	5	3.5	4	56	Yes	Yes

ICHD-II 1.1, 8.2	Number of patients		% pain relief long term
MO+	5		73%*
MO–	3		93%*

*Not sign.
[†] 13.12: Constant pain caused by compression, irritation or distortion of cranial nerves or upper cervical roots by structural lesions.
MD, missing data; MO+/–, with or without medication overuse at long-term follow-up.

Chapter 5

Table 4. Outcome data for all other patients

Patient	Baseline ICHD-II diagnosis*	VAS scores for pain pre-implantation actual/worst/least/mean				VAS scores for pain at 1 month actual/worst/least/mean				VAS scores for pain long-term actual/worst/least/mean				% pain relief long term	MO long-term	Redo long-term
4	4.8	8	8	1	7	1	2,5	1	1	1	7,5	1	5	0	Yes	No
6	5.2.2	MD	MD	MD	MD	MD	MD	MD	MD	MD	MD	MD	MD	52,5	No	MD
10	3.1.2, 1.6.1, A8.2	7	10	5	8	4	9	4	5,5	4,5	9	2,5	6	55	Yes	Yes
11	1.2.1, A8.2, 13.12	7	9	7	8	2	4	2	3	2	3	2	2,5	75	Yes	Yes
15	5.4	5,5	5,5	5,5	5,5	2	2	1	2	2	2	2	2	87,5	Yes	Yes
18	5.4	8	9	6	8	MD	MD	MD	MD	MD	MD	MD	MD	55	No	MD
20	NC	8	9	2,5	6	1	5	1	2	1	3	1	3	95	No	Yes
21	4.8	10	10	10	10	2	2	1	1,5	2,5	2,5	3	3	85	Yes	Yes
22	NC	8,5	9,5	6,5	8	3	6	2	2,5	MD	MD	MD	MD	15	Yes	MD
25	13.12, 1.2, A8.2	6,5	7	5	6,5	2	2	1	2	2	2	2	2	95	Yes	Yes

*1.2.1: Typical aura with migraine headache; 1.6.1: Probable migraine without aura; 3.1.2: Chronic cluster headache; 4.8: New daily persistent headache; 5.2.2: Chronic post-traumatic headache attributed to mild head injury; 5.4: Chronic headache attributed to whiplash injury; 13.12: Constant pain caused by compression, irritation or distortion of cranial nerves or upper cervical roots by structural lesions; A8.2: Medication overuse headache; NC, not classifiable; MD, missing data.

term follow-up. The overall aver- age percentage pain relief at long-term follow-up was 80%. There was no significant difference in percentage pain at long-term follow-up (see Table 3) between those patients with (n = 5) and those without medication overuse (n = 3) at long-term follow-up.

Other headache diagnoses

Diagnoses according to ICHD-II in the remaining 10 patients were diverse (see Table 4) and included new daily persistent headache (ICHD-II 4.8; n = 2), chronic post-traumatic headache attributed to mild head injury (ICHD-II 5.2.2; n = 1) and chronic headache attributed to whiplash injury (ICHD-II 5.4; n = 2). One patient suffered from chronic cluster headache, probable migraine and medication overuse headache (ICHD-II 3.1.2, 1.6.1 and A8.2; n = 1) Two patients had a combination of migraine with aura (ICHD-II 1.2.1) and ICHD-II 13.12 and two patients are not classifiable at present because they refused an indomethacin test. These 10 patients had an average follow-up of 27 months (range 9–68 months). All patients scored the efficacy at least good at 1 month's follow-up (n = 8, missing data in two). At long-term follow-up (missing data in three), only four of seven patients still scored the efficacy at least good. The patients experienced on average 62% pain relief at long-term follow-up (range 0–95%). At long-term follow-up six of seven patients would redo the intervention (missing data in three).

Discussion

The data presented suggest that for some subgroups of patients with relatively medically refractory headache ONS offers an effective, well-tolerated and comparatively safe approach to management. Certainly, in this very disabled group such a development would be welcome. The data provide support for the further study of ONS in migraine and caution investigators to monitor carefully for the potential effects of medication overuse when studying ONS. Perhaps more important, a cohort of patients with that may be described as Upper Cervical Neuropathic Pain (ICHD-II, 13.12). This finding is important, first, because the patients did well, and second, because such patients may not always come to the attention of neurology and headache specialists thinking about this new treatment modality. An important feature of our cohort has been the very careful phenotyping of the cases, including indomethacin testing, to provide as clear diagnoses as possible. ONS is a promising therapy for a range of patients, with challenges both to identify candidates and to conduct appropriately blinded randomized controlled trials.

Peripheral nerve stimulation, which is a minimally invasive and reversible procedure, is increasingly employed in the treatment of certain forms of chronic neuropathic pain and certainly preferred over nerve ablation procedures.[19] The mechanism of action is incompletely understood, but includes an inhibitory input within pain pathways, gate control of pain as well as modulation of neurotransmitters in the central nervous system.[19, 20] The technique of implantation of an occipital neurostimulator was pioneered by Weiner and Reed3 to treat patients with pain that had an occipital focus. Off-label use of ONS has been employed on a compassionate basis for highly disabled patients with intractable headache, suffering from occipital neuralgia[21], chronic migraine 5 or transformed migraine[22], chronic cluster headache[7, 8], hemicrania continua[13], post-traumatic headache and headache of C2 origin.[23] ONS is considered a minimally invasive procedure and safety data are good.[12] The rationale behind the technique in primary headache syndromes, such as migraine and cluster headache, is to modulate sensory traffic from the trigeminocervical complex[24, 25], either at the level of the second-order neurons[26, 27] or possibly in the thalamus.[5] Given the loss of spatial specificity at the level of the trigeminocervical complex, electrical stimulation of the occipital nerve may have an anti-nociceptive effect in the territory of the trigeminal as well as the occipital nerves. Interestingly, stimulation of the greater occipital nerve in the rat reduces calcitonin gene-related peptide in the jugular blood, which is a biomarker of inhibition of the trigeminal system.[28] In case of neuropathic pain in the occipital territory (ICHD-II 13.12), electrical stimulation of the sensory afferents may lead to suppression of Ad- and C-fibers at the level of the spinal dorsal horn.[29, 30]

We embarked on this retrospective study to try to identify subgroups of patients with medically refractory headache with an increased likelihood of responding to ONS. Response to an occipital nerve block certainly is not useful in predicting the therapeutic effect of ONS. [8, 10, 31] In this uncontrolled series all 44 patients had at least an occipital component to their head pain, and received uni- or bilateral ONS, mirroring the clinical distribution of the pain. At 1 month's follow-up post implantation, patient satisfaction was generally high and all patients would theoretically undergo the intervention again for the same indication. Given the mean duration of follow-up of 3 years and a total device time of almost 1600 months, the overall complication rate of two infections. However, at least one revision was needed in about 30% of patients because of technical problems, which included lead fracture, dislocation and connector current leakage. Some of these problems are due to the fact that the material used had not been designed for this purpose but for spinal cord stimulation. It is reassuring that not a single neurological deficit was created by the intervention. We only had two patients with a dislocated lead and not a single dislocation occurred after the technique was adapted by doing a medial incision, leaving loops at two stages and fixing the connector. These results are very favorable when compared with earlier results with lead dislocation in all patients after 3 years. [12] Twenty-six patients were phenotyped according to the ICHD-II criteria. At long-term follow-up 21 individuals indicated they experienced at least 50% pain relief. These 26 patients had a mean VAS reduction for 'average pain last week' of 4.7 at 1 month post implantation and of 3.4 at long-term follow-up. The overall satisfaction with the technique was high, except for three patients who had no pain relief at long-term follow-up. All three individuals, two migraine patients and one patient with new daily persistent headache, had ongoing medication overuse. When we compared available data from the 18 who were not phenotyped and the 26 who were, only few statistically significant differences were found, and these did not seem clinically important. For the rest of the discussion we speculate that our findings in the phenotyped patients are representative of the entire group. After sub analysis, two main groups of patients were identified, i.e. migraine without aura and occipital neuropathic pain, coded in the ICHD-II under 13.12 'Constant pain caused by compression, irritation or distortion of cranial nerves or upper cervical roots by structural lesions'. Even though both groups consisted of only eight patients, and thus statistical power is low, some significant differences were found. It appears that ICHD-II 13.12 patients had a higher percentage pain relief at long-term follow-up. This result is influenced by two migraine patients with ongoing medication overuse headache who experienced no pain relief at long-term follow-up and who indicated they would not redo the intervention at that time. Indeed, the presence/ persistence of medication overuse at long-term follow-up is associated with poor outcome in migraine patients, as the average pain relief for patients with medication overuse was much less than for those without a long-term follow-up. This finding is certainly consistent with the general concept that medication overuse renders migraine patients more resistant to prophylactic therapy. Thus, it appears that close monitoring of acute headache treatment is mandatory to ensure long-term benefit from the technique. Withdrawal of migraine patients from medication overuse is necessary prior to implantation, as it may account for a large part of the improvement by itself. These findings need to be corroborated in randomized, blinded and controlled trials, as a placebo effect, regression to the mean and spontaneous improvement certainly may play a role in the observed effect. A prospective daily headache diary would certainly be desirable in future studies to avoid recall bias.

Some individuals did not have long-term headache improvement after occipital neurostimulator implant, despite improvement in the temporary stimulator trial, as has previously been observed.12 Non-specific effects may have waned after permanent implantation. An important weakness of the study is that it is retrospective with regard to the pain aspects, although this is offset by the long-term follow-up and the careful approach to phenotyping the cases that has been employed. Due to the retrospective nature of the study, some data are missing. Fortunately, limited data are missing in the two main subgroups of patients, so that we are confident this does not affect the main conclusions of the study. Ideally, the questionnaires developed by the Belgian Pain Society would be validated for this kind of work.

Conclusion

Results of ONS for refractory headache are promising, although the concept of intractable headache itself needs to be refined further. The purpose of the definition of refractory must be clear, since the bar to a referral to an expert should be less than for a new therapy that is non-invasive vs. an invasive treatment. A number of issues need to be resolved to optimize ONS, including stimulus parameters, battery life, and the stimulator itself with regard to implantation techniques and associated side-effects, such as lead migration. An externally rechargeable battery would certainly be welcome. Moreover, patient selection criteria, as well as predictors for outcome, need to be further refined, and tested in clinical trials. Our retrospective study and a recent pilot study[23] generate the hypothesis that ICHD-II 13.12 may be an excellent indication for ONS, and a well-powered controlled trial would certainly be welcome. Careful clinical phenotyping will require close collaboration between pain specialists and neurologists, to assign diagnosis according to the ICHD-II. Many patients have been reclassified in this study, and it is clear, that multidisciplinary collaboration is essential for the scientific evaluation of ONS. In particular migraine patients need to be closely monitored for medication overuse, as is appears to be associated with poor long-term outcome in our study. ONS is promising and challenging for all concerned, although the prospect of finding therapies for our most disabled.

Chapter 5

References

1	Andlin-Sobocki P, Jonsson B, Wittchen HU, Olesen J. Cost of disorders of the brain in Europe. *Eur J Neurol*. 2005;12 Suppl 1:1-27.
2	Goadsby PJ, Schoenen J, Ferrari MD, Silberstein SD, Dodick D. Towards a definition of intractable headache for use in clinical practice and trials. *Cephalalgia*. 2006;26:1168-1170.
3	Weiner RL, Reed KL. Peripheral neurostimulation for control of intractable occipital neuralgia. *Neuromodulation*. 1999;2:217-221.
4	Headache classification subcommittee of the International Headache Society. The International Classification of Headache Disorders: 2nd edition *Cephalgia*. 2004;24:9-160.
5	Matharu MS, Bartsch T, Ward N, Frackowiak RS, Weiner R, Goadsby PJ. Central neuromodulation in chronic migraine patients with suboccipital stimulators: a PET study. *Brain*. 2004;127:220-230.
6	Afridi SK, Shields KG, Bhola R, Goadsby PJ. Greater occipital nerve injection in primary headache syndromes-- prolonged effects from a single injection. *Pain*. 2006;122:126-129.
7	Magis D, Allena M, Bolla M, De Pasqua V, Remacle JM, Schoenen J. Occipital nerve stimulation for drug-resistant chronic cluster headache: a prospective pilot study. *Lancet Neurol*. 2007;6:314-321.
8	Burns B, Watkins L, Goadsby PJ. Treatment of medically intractable cluster headache by occipital nerve stimulation: long-term follow-up of eight patients. *Lancet*. 2007;369:1099-1106.
9	Leone M. Deep brain stimulation in headache. *Lancet Neurol*. 2006;5:873-877.
10	Goadsby P, Dodick D, Saper J, Silberstein S. Occipital Nerve Stimulation (ONS) for Treatment of Intractable Chronic Migraine (ONSTIM). *Cephalalgia* 2009;29:133.
11	Schwedt TJ, Dodick DW, Trentman TL, Zimmerman RS. Occipital nerve stimulation for chronic cluster headache and hemicrania continua: pain relief and persistence of autonomic features. *Cephalalgia*. 2006;26:1025-1027.
12	Schwedt TJ, Dodick DW, Hentz J, Trentman TL, Zimmerman RS. Occipital nerve stimulation for chronic headache-- long-term safety and efficacy. *Cephalalgia*. 2007;27:153-157.
13	Burns B, Watkins L, Goadsby PJ. Treatment of hemicrania continua by occipital nerve stimulation with a bion device: long-term follow-up of a crossover study. *Lancet Neurol*. 2008;7:1001-1012.
14	Bartsch T, Paemeleire K, Goadsby PJ. Neurostimulation approaches to primary headache disorders. *Curr Opin Neurol*. 2009;22:262-268.
15	Paemeleire K, Van Buyten J, Van Buynder M, et al. Phenotype of patients responsive to suboccipital neurostimulation for refractory head pain. *Eur J Neurol*. 2008;15:10.
16	Silberstein SD, Olesen J, Bousser MG, et al. The International Classification of Headache Disorders, 2nd Edition (ICHD-II)--revision of criteria for 8.2 Medication-overuse headache. *Cephalalgia*. 2005;25:460-465.
17	Antonaci F, Pareja JA, Caminero AB, Sjaastad O. Chronic paroxysmal hemicrania and hemicrania continua. Parenteral indomethacin: the 'indotest'. *Headache*. 1998;38:122-128.
18	R FfSC. R: a language and environment for statistical computing. WWW document,http://www.r-project.org/.
19	Stojanovic MP. Stimulation methods for neuropathic pain control. *Curr Pain Headache Rep*. 2001;5:130-137.
20	Hanai F. Effect of electrical stimulation of peripheral nerves on neuropathic pain. *Spine (Phila Pa 1976)*. 2000;25:1886-1892.
21	Johnstone CS, Sundaraj R. Occipital nerve stimulation for the treatment of occipital neuralgia-eight case studies. *Neuromodulation*. 2006;9:41-47.
22	Popeney CA, Alo KM. Peripheral neurostimulation for the treatment of chronic, disabling transformed migraine. *Headache*. 2003;43:369-375.
23	Melvin EA, Jr., Jordan FR, Weiner RL, Primm D. Using peripheral stimulation to reduce the pain of C2-mediated occipital headaches: a preliminary report. *Pain Physician*. 2007;10:453-460.
24	Bartsch T, Goadsby PJ. Stimulation of the greater occipital nerve induces increased central excitability of dural afferent input. *Brain*. 2002;125:1496-1509.
25	Bartsch T, Goadsby PJ. Increased responses in trigeminocervical nociceptive neurons to cervical input after stimulation of the dura mater. *Brain*. 2003;126:1801-1813.
26	Piovesan EJ, Kowacs PA, Tatsui CE, Lange MC, Ribas LC, Werneck LC. Referred pain after painful stimulation of the greater occipital nerve in humans: evidence of convergence of cervical afferences on trigeminal nuclei. *Cephalalgia*. 2001;21:107-109.

27   Busch V, Jakob W, Juergens T, Schulte-Mattler W, Kaube H, May A. Functional connectivity between trigeminal and occipital nerves revealed by occipital nerve blockade and nociceptive blink reflexes. *Cephalalgia*. 2006;26:50-55.

28   Vincent MB, Ekman R, Edvinsson L, Sand T, Sjaastad O. Reduction of calcitonin gene-related peptide in jugular blood following electrical stimulation of rat greater occipital nerve. *Cephalalgia*. 1992;12:275-279.

29   Campbell JN, Taub A. Local analgesia from percutaneous electrical stimulation. A peripheral mechanism. *Arch Neurol*. 1973;28:347-350.

30   Melzack R, Wall PD. Pain mechanisms: a new theory. *Science*. 1965;150:971-979.

31   Schwedt TJ, Dodick DW, Trentman TL, Zimmerman RS. Response to occipital nerve block is not useful in predicting efficacy of occipital nerve stimulation. *Cephalalgia*. 2007;27:271-274.

We report our experience with DRG stimulation for the treatment of complex regional pain syndrome

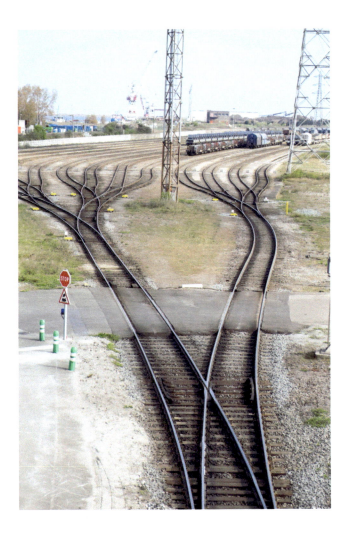

Chapter 6
Stimulation of Dorsal Root Ganglia for the Management of Complex Regional Pain Syndrome: A Prospective Case Series

Jean-Pierre Van Buyten [1], Iris Smet [1], Liong Liem [2], Marc Russo [3], Frank Huygen [4]

1 Multidisciplinary Pain Center, Algemeen Ziekenhuis Nikolaas, Sint-Niklaas, Belgium;
2 Sint Antonius Hospital, Nieuwegein, the Netherlands;
3 Hunter Pain Clinic, Broadmeadow, New South Wales, Australia;
4 Erasmus University, Rotterdam, the Netherlands

Abstract

Background:

Complex regional pain syndrome (CRPS) is a chronic and progressive pain condition usually involving the extremities and characterized by sensorimotor, vascular, and trophic changes. Spinal cord stimulation (SCS) is an effective intervention for this condition, but is hampered by the technical challenges associated with precisely directing stimulation to distal extremities. Dorsal root ganglia (DRG) may be more effective as a physiological target for electrical modulation due to recruitment of the primary sensory neurons that innervate the painful distal anatomical regions.

Methods:

Eleven subjects diagnosed with uni- or bilateral lower-extremity CRPS were recruited as part of a larger study involving chronic pain of heterogeneous etiologies. Quadripolar epidural leads of a newly developed neurostimulation system were placed near lumbar DRGs using conventional percutaneous techniques. The neurostimulators were trialed; 8 were successful and permanently implanted and programed to achieve optimal pain–paresthesia overlap.

Results:

All 8 subjects experienced some degree of pain relief and subjective improvement in function, as measured by multiple metrics. One month after implantation of the neurostimulator, there was significant reduction in average self-reported pain to 62% relative to baseline values. Pain relief persisted through 12 months in most subjects. In some subjects, edema and trophic skin changes associated with CRPS were also mitigated and function improved. Neuro- modulation of the DRG was able to provide excellent pain– paresthesia concordance in locations that are typically hard to target with traditional SCS, and the stimulation reduced the area of pain distributions.

Conclusions:

Neuromodulation of the DRG appears to be a promising option for relieving chronic pain and other symptoms associated with CRPS. The capture of discrete painful areas such as the feet, combined with stable paresthesia intensities independent of body position, suggests this stimulation modality may allow more selective and consistent targeting of painful areas than traditional SCS.

Key Words:
complex regional pain syndrome, dorsal root ganglion, spinal cord stimulation, neuromodulation, prospective case study

Chapter 6

Introduction

Complex regional pain syndrome (CRPS) is a pain disorder involving the extremities and is usually initiated after an injury, surgery, or vascular accident, although spontaneous development is also described. In addition to experiencing regional pain disproportionate to the inciting event,[1] patients with CRPS may experience sensory, vasomotor, sudomotor abnormalities, and motor/trophic changes.[2, 3] Muscle wasting can occur in the affected limb over time.[4] Fracture is the most common injury leading to CRPS, with upper extremities being affected more than lower extremities.[5]

According to the International Association for the Study of Pain (IASP), CRPS can be recognized as 2 distinct conditions: CRPS type I (formerly called reflex sympathetic dystrophy [RSD]) and CRPS type II (causalgia).[6] More recently, the clinical diagnostic criteria for CRPS, also known as the "Budapest criteria," have been revised. These describe CRPS as "an array of painful conditions that are characterized by a continuing regional pain that is seemingly disproportionate in time or degree to the usual course of any known trauma or other lesion. The pain is regional and usually has a distal predominance of abnormal sensory, motor, sudomotor, vasomotor, and/ or trophic findings. The syndrome shows variable progression over time."[7]

Epidemiological data are imprecise regarding CRPS due in part to historical changes in taxonomy (including RSD, causalgia, and algodystrophy[8]) and the misdiagnosis of early-stage CRPS as other disorders including normal post-traumatic processes,[9] but incidence rates may be approximately 5 to 25 cases per 100,000 person-years, with women at 4 times the risk of men. [2, 5, 10]

CRPS is thought to be initiated and maintained by a complex interaction of the sensorimotor, autonomic, and inflammatory systems. The pathophysiology involves peripheral, afferent, efferent, and central mechanisms. In the periphery, release of substance P and calcitonin gene-related peptide11 and a number of cytokines such as interleukin-6 and tumor necrosis factor-alpha12 contribute to neurogenic inflammation. Vasoconstriction appears to be under the influence of altered levels of endothelin-I and nitric oxide.[13] Skin biopsies from the affected limbs of patients diagnosed with CRPS-1 show degeneration of cutaneous nociceptors (reductions in C- and Ad-nerve endings in the epidermis[14]). As with other neuropathic pain conditions, sensitization of primary afferent, spinal, and/or supraspinal neurons occurs in CRPS.[15] This may indicate that maladaptive feedback loops and neuro- plasticity are established after the initiating insult. Additionally, although some patients may have experienced the stigma of perceived mental health issues, a recent review found no relationship between psycho- logical factors and the emergence of CRPS type 1.[16] It should be noted that psychological comorbidities such as depression are common as a result of chronic pain in general.[17] This also applies to CRPS. Spontaneous remission can occur in early stages,10 and best evidence suggests that early treatment may result in better outcomes,[18] as the percentage of subjects recovering from chronic or severe CRPS is low.[19] Treatment for CRPS typically involves an interdisciplinary approach.[20] The treatment for both types of CRPS is primarily aimed at alleviating pain and restoration of function with secondary goals of improving other signs and symptoms. Based on the predominant symptom, therapies could be focused on addressing the inflammation (free radical scavengers, bisphosphonates,[21, 22] and steroids), vasomotor disturbances (vasodilator therapies, including limited areas for sympathetic blocks [23, 24]), motor (baclofen[25]), and sensory (antineuropathic pain medication) abnormalities.[26, 27] Medical management typically includes pharmacological options in accordance with international guidelines for neuropathic pain [28] and physical therapy.[29] Good outcomes in CRPS include the reduction in pain, return of normal function to the affected limb, minimization of edema, and increased strength and range of motion at each of the affected joints.[30]

Spinal cord stimulation (SCS) is the recommended next-line intervention for patients with CRPS that is refractory to conventional approaches,[2, 4, 31, 32] based on the available evidence.33 SCS has been successfully applied since 1967 as a treatment modality for the management of chronic, intractable pain in the trunk, and/or limbs.[34] Mechanisms of SCS are based upon the gate control theory in which the non-noxious SCS paresthesias, carried via large, rapidly conducting nerve fibers, inhibit the input from small-diameter pain fibers.[35] Specific to CRPS, SCS may relieve its non-nociceptive pain by increasing GABAergic activity in the dorsal columns, thereby reducing sensory excitation from the periphery and by increasing peripheral vasodilation.[36]

Spinal cord stimulation has been demonstrated to improve CRPS pain and quality of life outcomes in a randomized controlled trial, and to be cost effective in the first 2 years after implantation.[37-39] However, comparing its benefit against conventional therapy could not demonstrate a statistically significant difference at 5 years.[40] Others report that 56% of CRPS patients have 50% pain relief at an average of 4.4 years post implant [41] and that approximately 40% of patients have better than 30% pain relief through 11 years.[42] Limitations experienced are lead breakage and migration, loss of coverage (stimulation-induced paresthesias), or partial coverage of the pain area.[43, 44] Pathophysiological changes in the DRG may be a contributory factor to the development of CRPS, and therefore, stimulation of this target may have beneficial effects on the painful symptoms associated with CRPS. Prospectively identifying which CRPS patients will respond successfully to SCS remains difficult. One obstacle to optimum results with SCS is to achieve optimal pain–paresthesia overlap in distal extremities while simultaneously limiting the side effect of extraneous stimulation.[45, 46] SCS is acknowledged to provide incomplete or inconsistent coverage of some areas, including the low back, buttocks, feet, groin, pelvis, and neck.[47] Furthermore, SCS systems are susceptible to postural effects due to the potential for lead movement in the epidural space.[48, 49] Variations in the intensity of neurostimulation due to body position are a problem because positional changes may result in over- or under- stimulation, which can lead to frequent compensatory manual programming adjustments. Therefore, alternative neuromodulatory approaches may be needed. Dorsal root ganglion (DRG) stimulation, in which the electrodes are placed adjacent relatively immobile spinal structures and activate highly specific sensory neurons, has shown promise for precisely steering pain-mitigating paresthesias into hard-to-reach locations.[50-53] This report describes the effects of DRG stimulation on CRPS symptoms in a small prospective cohort. It was hypothesized that this stimulation modality would achieve good pain–paresthesia overlap and that meaningful pain relief would be realized.

Methods

This study was conducted at 4 pain management clinics or hospitals in Europe and Australia under local ethical committee approval and with full informed consent of the subjects. Standard clinical diagnostic criteria for CRPS were employed (Budapest criteria for clinical use [7, 18, 30]): chronic pain that is disproportionate to the original injury and cannot be explained by another diagnosis, with the presence of at least 3 symptoms and at least 2 signs among sensory, vasomotor, sudomotor/ edema, and motor/trophic categories.[7, 18] Subjects were part of a larger prospective, open-label, single-arm clinical trial involving DRG stimulation for the treatment of chronic pain; this study has been described previously.[52, 53] Briefly, after baseline assessments, subjects were implanted with the AxiumTM Neurostimulator System (Spinal Modulation, Inc., Menlo Park, CA, U.S.A.) with quadripolar percutaneous leads placed near the DRG relevant to their pain distribution (Figure 1). If the trial period was successful, as defined by relief of 50% or more of overall pain, subjects received a fully implantable stimulator after approximately 1 week without stimulation. Clinical follow-ups occurred at 1 week, 1 month, 5 weeks, 2, 3, 6, and 12 months post implant and collected outcome measures across domains recommended by the IMMPACT group for multidimensional evaluations in pain clinical studies.54 At all time points, overall pain and pain specific to leg and foot distributions were assessed via a 100-mm visual analog scale (VAS) in which 0 mm indicated no pain and 100 mm indicated the worst imaginable pain. The Brief Pain Inventory (Short Form, BPISF)55 was used to further assess the impact of pain, mood was assessed with the Profile of Mood States (Short Form, POMS),56 and quality of life was assessed with the EuroQOL five dimensions' questionnaire (EQ-5D-3L).57 Safety out- comes (frequency of adverse events [AEs]) were tracked throughout the study. Trends are expressed in this report as means ± SEM or as percentages of baseline values, and hypothesis testing used 2-tailed t-tests with significance levels set at 0.05. Qualitative outcomes are also reported to provide context and clinical relevance.

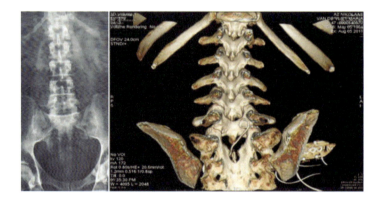

Figure 1: Anterior–Posterior (AP) view of leads implanted at right L4 and L5 dorsal root ganglia (DRGs) (left). 3-D reconstruction of a lead at L5 DRG using a computed tomography (CT) scan (right).

Results

Eleven subjects with CRPS were recruited and trialed with the DRG neuromodulation system. Two subjects reported < 50% improvement in their pain relief, whereas 1 subject had 100% pain relief in 1 foot and no pain relief in the other.

The average age of the 8 subjects (6 women and 2 men) with successful trial stimulation was 43.9 years (± 5.6; range: 18 to 65). At baseline, their overall pain was 77.9 (± 4.2) mm. During the trial period, these subjects reported a minimum of 50% pain relief; the average pain with trial stimulation was 14.0 (± 4.2) mm, an 81.9% reduction relative to baseline. Stimulation was discontinued at the end of the trial phase for about a week. During this period, the average pain rating rebounded to 73.8 (± 4.9) mm, which was statistically indistinguishable from baseline (P > 0.05). All 8 subjects received a permanently implanted neurostimulator (INS). One week after subjects received the INS (week 1), subjects reported that their average overall pain was reduced to 27.1 (± 7.6) mm, which represented an average 65.2% (± 10.3%) decrease from baseline (P < 0.001). At 1 month, the average pain was 30.0 (± 10.0) mm, a decrease of 62.1% relative to baseline (P < 0.005). Stimulation was temporarily suspended after the 1-month assessment to verify intrasubject effectiveness. After a week without stimulation (week 5), subjects reported that their overall pain returned to 55.6 (± 12.7) mm, which was not statistically significantly different from baseline (P > 0.05). At this point, 1 subject's INS were explanted due to unsatisfactory pain relief. At 3 months post-implant (n = 7), the average overall pain rating was 26.1 (± 11.6) mm (P < 0.001), a 68.4% (± 13.0%) decrease from baseline. At 6 months post-implant, average pain was 29.4 (± 11.3) mm, a 63.1% (± 13.2%) reduction from baseline (P < 0.005). At 12 months, subjects reported an overall pain of 30.3 (± 12.7) mm, a 61.7% (± 16.4%) decrease from baseline (P < 0.05), and 5 of the 7 subjects (71.4%) had greater than or equal to 50% pain relief. Similar patterns of responsiveness were observed for the foot- (n = 8) and leg-specific (n = 7) pain scores. These data are depicted in Figure 2. Both foot pain and leg pain were significantly lower with active stimulation at all follow-up time points compared with the baseline (ps < 0.05). At 12 months, 6 of the 7 subjects with foot pain (85.7%) and 4 of the 5 subjects with leg pain (80.0%) had greater than or equal to 50% pain relief in those regions.

With respect to secondary end points, the BPISF revealed statistically significant reductions relative to baseline at the 12-month follow-up time points in the pain severity and pain interference domains. Quality of life improved, as reflected in EQ-5D-3L VAS and utility index scores at 12 months, and this instrument's pain– discomfort dimension also indicated a reduction in pain at 12 months. Mood disturbance was decreased over the course of the study, and significant improvements were identified across tension, depression, and anger domains. These secondary endpoint data are presented in Table 1. As illustrated by the exemplar subject in Figure 3, the distribution of painful areas generally shrank after the initiation of stimulation and remained stable over time and across body positions. Exact pain–paresthesia concordance was often achieved, even to the degree of recruiting a single toe.

Table 1. Statistically Significant Improvements from Baseline were Observed at the 12-Month Follow-Up in All Secondary Endpoint Comparisons

	Baseline (n = 8)	12 months (n = 7)
BPISF		
Pain severity	6.9 ± 0.4	3.2 ± 1.2*
Pain interference	7.3 ± 0.6	3.4 ± 1.3*
EQ-5D-3L		
VAS	39.9 ± 9.5	69.3 ± 11.6*
Utility index	0.25 ± 0.08 (n = 6)	0.70 ± 0.10* (n = 6)
POMS[†]		
Tension	8.3 ± 1.3	3.9 ± 1.2*
Depression	8.4 ± 1.7	2.6 ± 1.6*
Anger	7.6 ± 1.6	2.0 ± 1.1*
Total mood disturbance score	37.3 ± 5.4	10.4 ± 7.3*

*$P < 0.05$ relative to the baseline score of that dimension.
[†]Three other subscales, vigor, fatigue, and confusion improved from the baseline but did not reach significance.

Some subjects showed obvious neurovascular changes and improvement in mobility. For example, a subject with severe erysipelas in his left leg and foot at baseline (Figure 4A) reported reduced swelling

Chapter 6

and improved coloration in the affected foot after 1 month (Figure 4B). By 6 months post-implant, the swelling had entirely resolved (Figure 4C). The subject reported that his function was "100% improved" and rated his quality of life after the initiation of INS as "100 out of 100." Another subject reported that, in addition to pain relief, her foot also regained normal flexion parameters and she regained better mobility, especially in climbing stairs. A third subject evidenced better mobility by being able to walk around the house with only 1 crutch. Interestingly, 2 subjects reported bilateral CRPS in both their lower limbs. One of those subjects reported nearly complete pain reduction in both feet; the other subject had excellent improvement in 1 limb, but poor outcome in the second limb.

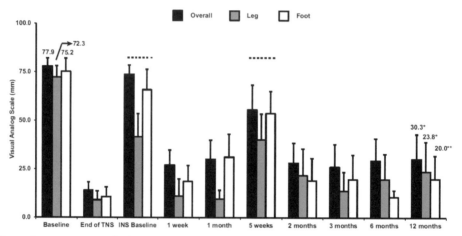

Figure 2: Average overall, leg, and foot pain rating during the trial and implantation phases of treatment with the dorsal root ganglia (DRG) stimulation unit. Error bars indicated standard error of the mean. The dotted bar represents time points when stimulation was turned off (1 week after the end of the trial period and at week 5) to evaluate pain in the absence of stimulation. *P < 0.05 and **P<0.005.

Eleven AEs were reported in 4 subjects (not related to the device – 8, possibly related – 2, definitely related – 1); 3 were classified as mild, 5 as moderate, and 3 as severe. One of the AEs, discomfort associated with stimulation, was resolved by reprograming. No lead revisions were required. A complete list of AEs can be found in Table 2. Two serious AEs (prolonged hospital stay and lack of paresthesia coverage), both unrelated to the device, were reported in 2 different subjects. The former SAE was due to moderate pain experienced by the subject resulting in hospitalization (lack of caregivers at home) whereas the latter SAE was resolved through lead revision.

Discussion

All 8 subjects implanted with a DRG neurostimulator for CRPS reported some pain relief. Good results (greater than or equal to 50% pain relief in the foot) were reported after 12 months of treatment for 6 of the 8 subjects. This responder rate is similar to or better than reported outcomes with SCS for CRPS38-42 and confirms DRG stimulation as a viable and effective intervention for this difficult pain condition. Mechanisms of action for DRG-mediated pain relief involve modulation of primary sensory neurons.58 Pathophysiologic alterations of the primary sensory neurons are generally thought to contribute to the development and maintenance of chronic or intractable pain[59] examples of such alterations may include abnormal expression and regulation of ion channels. Previous reports have implicated the DRG in the development and maintenance of chronic pain,[60, 61] and electrical field stimulation has been demonstrated to alter the excitability of DRG neurons.[62]

Improvements in perfusion and trophic changes in the affected limbs were observed in some subjects, as has been reported in SCS.[4] With SCS, it is theorized that vascular changes occur due to the antidromic activation of sensory afferents, which in turn releases vasodilatory peptides[36]; it is likely that this mechanism is also applicable to DRG stimulation, in which primary sensory neurons are activated. With further research, it could be demonstrated that DRG stimulation may activate a reflex arc involving GABAergic interneurons that project to the sympathetic premotor neurons in the intermediolateral cell column, as has been theorized to underlie good CRPS outcomes with SCS.[36]

This study may be underpowered for some measures, and as with any small sample, it may not be possible to generalize the results of this cohort to the larger CRPS population. However, it should be noted that trends toward improvements were noted in other measures (back- and leg-specific pain, pain intensity, quality of life, and mood). Because converging results across multiple outcome measures (according to pain study design recommendations[54]) were obtained, the conclusions may be more robust.

No lead migration was reported through the 12- month follow-up in the 7 subjects, in contrast to the 11 lead repositioning's that were required in 24 CRPS patients with SCS over the course of 5 years[40] or the annual mean intervention rate of 7% to 13% due to lead migration in another long-term study of CRPS patients with SCS.[42] Another striking outcome of this study was the demonstration of the specificity of pain– paresthesia overlap in distal extremities, to the extent of being able to achieve coverage of individual toes. Additionally, stimulation remained stable both over time and across different body positions. The precision and stability of the paresthesias produced with DRG stimulation has also been reported in a larger sample.[53] With traditional SCS, leads in the epidural space may change position in response to body movements or altered posture; as the leads move subtly closer to or farther from the dorsal columns, the perceived stimulation may become more or less intense.[45, 63] In DRG neurostimulation, electrodes are closer to the target, allowing more focused neurostimulation, and are far less likely to shift due to movement or postures. Given the localized nature of CRPS symptoms, DRG stimulation may thus be a more attractive intervention than SCS.

Chapter 6

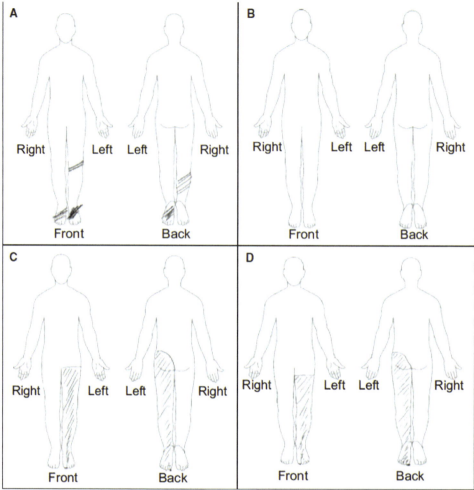

Figure 3: Pain distribution at (A) baseline and (B) week 1 of a representative subject with good treatment response. At 12 months, self-reported paresthesia distributions were identical whether the subject was (C) upright or (D) supine.

Table 2. List of Adverse Events, their Severity, and Relationship to the Device

No.	Description	Severity	Relationship to Device
1	Prolonged hospital stay	Mild	Not related
2	Pain in right hip	Moderate	Not related
3	Cellulitis in lower legs	Moderate	Not related
4	Ulcer in right foot	Moderate	Not related
5	Knee replacement	Moderate	Not related
6	Pain in left buttock over, IPG implant	Severe	Possibly related
7	Intermittent cramping in right calf	Severe	Possibly related
8	Nausea	Mild	Not related
9	Pain in hand and forearm	Mild	Not related
10	Discomfort from stimulation	Moderate	Definitely related
11	Increased foot pain	Severe	Not related

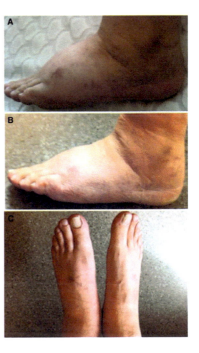

Figure 4: The neurovascular symptoms in the affected limb of 1 subject with good pain relief were greatly reduced from baseline.
(A) to 1 month (B) and 6 months (C). At 6 months, the subject reported that function was "100% improved."

Conclusions

Although results were mixed, all subjects had some pain relief and 3-quarters of the subjects in this prospective cohort of DRG stimulation experienced better than 50% pain relief in addition to improvements in mood and quality of life. Some subjects reported improved mobility and showed remission in some sympathetically maintained symptoms such as swelling and discoloration. Qualitatively, subjects were enthusiastic. This establishes DRG stimulation as a promising emerging therapy in the application of CRPS for otherwise intractable cases.

Chapter 6

References

1   Stanton-Hicks M, Janig W, Hassenbusch S, Haddox JD, Boas R, Wilson P. Reflex sympathetic dystrophy: changing concepts and taxonomy. *Pain*. 1995;63:127-133.
2   van Eijs F, Stanton-Hicks M, Van Zundert J, et al. Evidence-based interventional pain medicine according to clinical diagnoses. 16. Complex regional pain syndrome. *Pain Pract*. 2011;11:70-87.
3   Harden RN. Complex regional pain syndrome. *Br J Anaesth*. 2001;87:99-106.
4   Stanton-Hicks M. Complex regional pain syndrome: manifestations and the role of neurostimulation in its management. *J Pain Symptom Manage*. 2006;31:S20-24.
5   de Mos M, de Bruijn AG, Huygen FJ, Dieleman JP, Stricker BH, Sturkenboom MC. The incidence of complex regional pain syndrome: a population-based study. *Pain*. 2007;129:12-20.
6   International Association for the Study of Pain I, ed. *Classification of Chronic Pain: Descriptions of Chronic Pain Syndromes and Definitions of Pain Terms, 2nd ed. (Revised).*
, Washington DC: IASP Press;; 1994.
7   Harden RN, Bruehl S, Stanton-Hicks M, Wilson PR. Proposed new diagnostic criteria for complex regional pain syndrome. *Pain Med*. 2007;8:326-331.
8   Alvarez-Lario B, Aretxabala-Alcibar I, Alegre-Lopez J, Alonso-Valdivielso JL. Acceptance of the different denominations for reflex sympathetic dystrophy. *Ann Rheum Dis*. 2001;60:77-79.
9   Schurmann M, Gradl G, Andress HJ, Furst H, Schildberg FW. Assessment of peripheral sympathetic nervous function for diagnosing early post-traumatic complex regional pain syndrome type I. *Pain*. 1999;80:149-159.
10 Sandroni P, Benrud-Larson LM, McClelland RL, Low PA. Complex regional pain syndrome type I: incidence and prevalence in Olmsted county, a population-based study. *Pain*. 2003;103:199-207.
11 Marinus J, Moseley GL, Birklein F, et al. Clinical features and pathophysiology of complex regional pain syndrome. *Lancet Neurol*. 2011;10:637-648.
12 Huygen FJ, De Bruijn AG, De Bruin MT, Groeneweg JG, Klein J, Zijlstra FJ. Evidence for local inflammation in complex regional pain syndrome type 1. *Mediators Inflamm*. 2002;11:47-51.
13 Groeneweg JG, Huygen FJ, Heijmans-Antonissen C, Niehof S, Zijlstra FJ. Increased endothelin-1 and diminished nitric oxide levels in blister fluids of patients with intermediate cold type complex regional pain syndrome type 1. *BMC Musculoskelet Disord*. 2006;7:91.
14 Kharkar S, Venkatesh YS, Grothusen JR, Rojas L, Schwartzman RJ. Skin biopsy in complex regional pain syndrome: case series and literature review. *Pain Physician*. 2012;15:255-266.
15 Schwartzman RJ, Alexander GM, Grothusen J. Pathophysiology of complex regional pain syndrome. *Expert Rev Neurother*. 2006;6:669-681.
16 Beerthuizen A, van 't Spijker A, Huygen FJ, Klein J, de Wit R. Is there an association between psychological factors and the Complex Regional Pain Syndrome type 1 (CRPS1) in adults? A systematic review. *Pain*. 2009;145:52-59.
17 Tunks ER, Crook J, Weir R. Epidemiology of chronic pain with psychological comorbidity: prevalence, risk, course, and prognosis. *Can J Psychiatry*. 2008;53:224-234.
18 Harden RN, Oaklander AL, Burton AW, et al. Complex regional pain syndrome: practical diagnostic and treatment guidelines, 4th edition. *Pain Med*. 2013;14:180-229.

19 de Mos M, Huygen FJ, van der Hoeven-Borgman M, Dieleman JP, Ch Stricker BH, Sturkenboom MC. Outcome of the complex regional pain syndrome. *Clin J Pain*. 2009;25:590-597.
20 Turner-Stokes L, Goebel A, Guideline Development G. Complex regional pain syndrome in adults: concise guidance. *Clin Med (Lond)*. 2011;11:596-600.
21 Manicourt DH, Brasseur JP, Boutsen Y, Depreseux G, Devogelaer JP. Role of alendronate in therapy for posttraumatic complex regional pain syndrome type I of the lower extremity. *Arthritis Rheum*. 2004;50:3690-3697.
22 Robinson JN, Sandom J, Chapman PT. Efficacy of pamidronate in complex regional pain syndrome type I. *Pain Med*. 2004;5:276-280.
23 Cepeda MS, Carr DB, Lau J. Local anesthetic sympathetic blockade for complex regional pain syndrome. *Cochrane Database Syst Rev*. 2005:CD004598.
24 Price DD, Long S, Wilsey B, Rafii A. Analysis of peak magnitude and duration of analgesia produced by local anesthetics injected into sympathetic ganglia of complex regional pain syndrome patients. *Clin J Pain*. 1998;14:216-226.
25 van Rijn MA, Munts AG, Marinus J, et al. Intrathecal baclofen for dystonia of complex regional pain syndrome. *Pain*. 2009;143:41-47.

26   Tran DQ, Duong S, Bertini P, Finlayson RJ. Treatment of complex regional pain syndrome: a review of the evidence. *Can J Anaesth*. 2010;57:149-166.
27   Perez RS, Zollinger PE, Dijkstra PU, et al. Evidence based guidelines for complex regional pain syndrome type 1. *BMC Neurol*. 2010;10:20.
28   Attal N, Cruccu G, Baron R, et al. EFNS guidelines on the pharmacological treatment of neuropathic pain: 2009 revision. *Eur J Neurol*. 2010.
29   Daly AE, Bialocerkowski AE. Does evidence support physiotherapy management of adult Complex Regional Pain Syndrome Type One? A systematic review. *Eur J Pain*. 2009;13:339-353.
30   Harden RN, Bruehl S, Perez RS, et al. Development of a severity score for CRPS. *Pain*. 2010;151:870-876.
31   van Eijs F, Geurts JW, Van Zundert J, et al. Spinal cord stimulation in complex regional pain syndrome type I of less than 12-month duration. *Neuromodulation*. 2012;15:144-150; discussion 150.
32   Stanton-Hicks MD, Burton AW, Bruehl SP, et al. An updated interdisciplinary clinical pathway for CRPS: report of an expert panel. *Pain Pract*. 2002;2:1-16.
33   Van Zundert J, Hartrick C, Patijn J, Huygen F, Mekhail N, van Kleef M. Evidence-based interventional pain medicine according to clinical diagnoses. *Pain Pract*. 2011;11:423-429.
34   Shealy CN, Taslitz N, Mortimer JT, Becker DP. Electrical inhibition of pain: experimental evaluation. *Anesth Analg*. 1967;46:299-305.
35   Melzack R, Wall PD. Pain mechanisms: a new theory. *Science*. 1965;150:971-979.
36   Prager JP. What does the mechanism of spinal cord stimulation tell us about complex regional pain syndrome? *Pain Med*. 2010;11:1278-1283.
37   Kemler MA, Furnee CA. Economic evaluation of spinal cord stimulation for chronic reflex sympathetic dystrophy. *Neurology*. 2002;59:1203-1209.
38   Kemler MA, De Vet HC, Barendse GA, Van Den Wildenberg FA, Van Kleef M. The effect of spinal cord stimulation in patients with chronic reflex sympathetic dystrophy: two years' follow-up of the randomized controlled trial. *Ann Neurol*. 2004;55:13-18.
39   Kemler MA, Barendse GA, van Kleef M, et al. Spinal cord stimulation in patients with chronic reflex sympathetic dystrophy. *N Engl J Med*. 2000;343:618-624.

40   Kemler MA, de Vet HC, Barendse GA, van den Wildenberg FA, van Kleef M. Effect of spinal cord stimulation for chronic complex regional pain syndrome Type I: five-year final follow-up of patients in a randomized controlled trial. *J Neurosurg*. 2008;108:292-298.
41   Sears NC, Machado AG, Nagel SJ, et al. Long-term outcomes of spinal cord stimulation with paddle leads in the treatment of complex regional pain syndrome and failed back surgery syndrome. *Neuromodulation*. 2011;14:312-318; discussion 318.
42   Geurts JW, Smits H, Kemler MA, Brunner F, Kessels AG, van Kleef M. Spinal cord stimulation for complex regional pain syndrome type I: a prospective cohort study with long-term follow-up. *Neuromodulation*. 2013;16:523-529; discussion 529.
43   Barolat G, Schwartzman R, Woo R. Epidural spinal cord stimulation in the management of reflex sympathetic dystrophy. *Stereotact Funct Neurosurg*. 1989;53:29-39.
44   Grabow TS, Tella PK, Raja SN. Spinal cord stimulation for complex regional pain syndrome: an evidence-based medicine review of the literature. *Clin J Pain*. 2003;19:371-383.
45   Holsheimer J, Khan YN, Raza SS, Khan EA. Effects of electrode positioning on perception threshold and paresthesia coverage in spinal cord stimulation. *Neuromodulation*. 2007;10:34-41.
46   Lee D, Gillespie E, Bradley K. Dorsal column steerability with dual parallel leads using dedicated power sources: a computational model. *J Vis Exp*. 2011.
47   Stuart RM, Winfree CJ. Neurostimulation techniques for painful peripheral nerve disorders. *Neurosurg Clin N Am*. 2009;20:111-120, vii-viii.
48   Cameron T, Alo KM. Effects of posture on stimulation parameters in spinal cord stimulation. *Neuromodulation*. 1998;1:177-183.
49   Schultz DM, Webster L, Kosek P, Dar U, Tan Y, Sun M. Sensor-driven position-adaptive spinal cord stimulation for chronic pain. *Pain Physician*. 2012;15:1-12.
50   Haque R, Winfree CJ. Spinal nerve root stimulation. *Neurosurg Focus*. 2006;21:E4.
51   Lynch PJ, McJunkin T, Eross E, Gooch S, Maloney J. Case report: successful epiradicular peripheral nerve stimulation of the C2 dorsal root ganglion for postherpetic neuralgia. *Neuromodulation*. 2011;14:58-61; discussion 61.

Chapter 6

52   Deer TR, Grigsby E, Weiner RL, Wilcosky B, Kramer JM. A prospective study of dorsal root ganglion stimulation for the relief of chronic pain. *Neuromodulation*. 2013;16:67-71; discussion 71-62.
53   Liem L, Russo M, Huygen FJ, et al. A multicenter, prospective trial to assess the safety and performance of the spinal modulation dorsal root ganglion neurostimulator system in the treatment of chronic pain. *Neuromodulation*. 2013;16:471-482; discussion 482.
54   Dworkin RH, Turk DC, Peirce-Sandner S, et al. Considerations for improving assay sensitivity in chronic pain clinical trials: IMMPACT recommendations. *Pain*. 2012;153:1148-1158.
55   Tan G, Jensen MP, Thornby JI, Shanti BF. Validation of the Brief Pain Inventory for chronic nonmalignant pain. *J Pain*. 2004;5:133-137.
56   Curran S, Andrykowski M, Studts J. Short form of the Profile of Mood States (POMS-SF): psychometric information. *Psychol Assess*. 1995;7:80-83.
57   EuroQol Group T. EuroQol--a new facility for the measurement of health-related quality of life. . *Health Policy*. 1990;16:199-208.
58   Hogan QH. Labat lecture: the primary sensory neuron: where it is, what it does, and why it matters. *Reg Anesth Pain Med*. 2010;35:306-311.
59   Campbell JN, Meyer RA. Mechanisms of neuropathic pain. *Neuron*. 2006;52:77-92.
60   Sapunar D, Kostic S, Banozic A, Puljak L. Dorsal root ganglion - a potential new therapeutic target for neuropathic pain. *J Pain Res*. 2012;5:31-38.
61   Van Zundert J, Patijn J, Kessels A, Lame I, van Suijlekom H, van Kleef M. Pulsed radiofrequency adjacent to the cervical dorsal root ganglion in chronic cervical radicular pain: a double blind sham controlled randomized clinical trial. *Pain*. 2007;127:173-182.
62   Koopmeiners AS, Mueller S, Kramer J, Hogan QH. Effect of electrical field stimulation on dorsal root ganglion neuronal function. *Neuromodulation*. 2013;16:304-311; discussion 310-301.
63   He J, Barolat G, Holsheimer J, Struijk JJ. Perception threshold and electrode position for spinal cord stimulation. *Pain*. 1994;59:55-63.

We evaluated whether stimulation of the medial branch restores dynamic stability of the back.

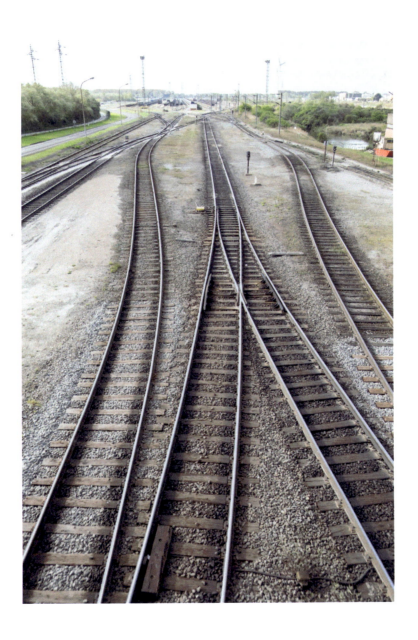

Chapter 7
Chronic Low Back Pain: Restoration of Dynamic Stability

Kristiaan Deckers, MD[1]; Kris De Smedt, MD[2]; Jean-Pierre van Buyten, MD[3]; Iris Smet, MD[3]; Sam Eldabe, MD[4]; Ashish Gulve, MD[4]; Ganesan Baranidharan, MD[5]; José de Andrès, MD, PhD[6]; Chris Gilligan, MD[7]; Kristen Jaax, MD, PhD[8]; Jan Pieter Heemels, MS[8]; Peter Crosby, MS[8]

[1] Department of Physical Medicine and Rehabilitation, GZA Hospitals, Antwerpen, Belgium;
[2] Department of Neurosurgery, GZA Hospitals, Antwerpen, Belgium;
[3] Multidisciplinary Pain Centre, AZ Nikolaas, Sint Niklaas, Belgium;
[4] Department of Pain and Anesthesia, The James Cook University Hospital, Middlesbrough, UK;
[5] Leeds Pain and Neuromodulation Centre, Leeds Teaching Hospitals NHS Trust, Leeds, UK;
[6] Anesthesia Critical Care and Pain Management, General University Hospital, Valencia, Spain;
[7] Massachusetts General Hospital, Center for Pain Medicine, Boston, USA; and
[8] Mainstay Medical Limited, Swords, Ireland

Neuromodulation. 2015;18:478-486

Abstract

Objectives:
Electrical stimulation for multifidus muscle contraction is a novel approach for treating chronic low back pain (CLBP). A multicenter, open-label feasibility study investigated this modality in patients with continuing CLBP despite medical management and no prior back surgery and no known pathological cause of CLBP.

Methods:
Twenty-six patients with continuing CLBP despite physical therapy and medication were implanted with commercially- available implantable pulse generators and leads positioned adjacent to the medial branch of the dorsal ramus as it crosses the L3 transverse process such that electrical stimulation resulted in contraction of the lumbar multifidus (LM) muscle. Patients self-administered stimulation twice daily for 20 min. Low back pain (VAS), Oswestry Disability Index (ODI) and Quality of Life (EQ-5D) scores were collected at three and five months and compared to baseline. Stimulation was withdrawn between months 4 and 5 to test durability of effect.

Results:
At three months, 74% of patients met or exceeded the minimally important change (MIC) in VAS and 63% for disability. QoL improved in 84% of patients (N = 19) and none got worse. Five of the 11 patients on disability for CLBP (45%) resumed work by three months. Half the patients reported ≥50% VAS reduction by month 5. Twenty-one lead migration events occurred in 13 patients, of which 7 patients are included in the efficacy cohort.

Conclusions:
Episodic stimulation to induce LM contraction can reduce CLBP and disability, improve quality of life and enable return to work. A dedicated lead design to reduce risk of migration is required.

Keywords:
Low back pain, motor control, multifidus, quality of life, stimulation

Chapter 7

Introduction

Chronic Low Back Pain

Chronic low back pain (CLBP) is a widespread condition, with best estimates suggesting that lifetime prevalence is around 23% [1]. Patients with CLBP usually suffer impaired quality of life (QoL) and score significantly higher on scales for depression, anxiety and sleep disorders. [2] The resulting economic impact of days lost from work, disability benefits and health resource utilization are estimated to be as high as 1.7% of GDP in some countries. [3]

Although in some patients a specific pathology can be identified as the cause of CLBP, for many there is no clear association between identifiable pathology on imaging and their CLBP symptoms. [4]

Role of the Lumbar Multifidus

The major muscle contributing to local stability of the lumbar spine is the lumbar multifidus [5-7] (LM) (Fig. 1) which has a unique structure ideally suited for its stabilizing role. Functionally, the LM is divided into deep, intermediate and superficial fibers, with deep fibers spanning two vertebral segments and functioning tonically, and intermediate and superficial fibers spanning three to five levels and functioning phasically. [8, 9] This arrangement makes the deep fibers of the LM anatomically and biomechanically well suited both to provide feedback regarding the position of the spine (proprioception) and, in turn, provide stabilization of the spine.

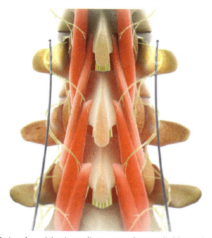

Figure 1: Lead positioning adjacent to the medial branch as it crosses the L3 transverse process. Muscles shown in image are the deep fascicles of the lumbar multifidi (LM).

Lumbar Multifidus Reflex Inhibition

Pain in a joint has been shown to reduce neural drive to the muscles that stabilize the joint, which is known as reflex inhibition.

Reflex inhibition is commonly observed in the knee where it is referred to as Arthrogenic Muscle Inhibition. [10] This phenomenon is due to an inhibitory process involving afferent discharge from mechanoreceptors or nociceptors in the joint structures. [11] Experimental evidence in animal models has demonstrated that local injury to spinal structures, including experimentally induced intervertebral disc degeneration and nerve root injury, leads to reduction in neural drive to the LM, evidenced by reduced electrical activity on electromyography (EMG). [12, 13]

Reduction in LM EMG activity has been observed in humans with both induced pain studies [14, 15] and studies of patients with acute or chronic LBP. [16, 17] Ultrasound imaging evidence of reduced neural drive in LBP patients includes diminished cross sectional area with contraction[18], reduced ability to cause a muscle thickness change on command [19], and altered contraction patterns with changes in posture. [20] MRI studies suggest that patients suffering from chronic LBP are more likely to have atrophy of the LM com- pared to healthy controls. [21] Further, LM atrophy can be seen easily and reliably on MRI [22] and often occurs within days of onset of new LBP. [23] Hodges et al. demonstrated that the parts of the muscle that overlay an injured segment, such as a disc lesion, are most affected by atrophy. Localization to a single vertebral level suggests that atrophy may specifically involve the deeper fibers responsible for spine stabilization; this may be related to greater sensitivity of the deep fibers to inhibition or the relatively higher proportion of type I muscle fibers in these deep layers. [13]

Persistent Motor Control Impairment Leads to Chronic Low Back Pain

Although reflex inhibition may be protective at first, if not reversed it may evolve into a self-sustained Motor Control Impairment (MCI). [24, 25] The patient's inability to effectively recruit the affected muscle can lead to muscle atrophy[13, 23], maladaptive recruitment patterns [26], distorted proprioception [27] and accelerated muscle fatigue [28] resulting in impaired dynamic spinal stability and loading. The resulting inability to maintain the spinal joints within a pain-free range of motion leads to increased susceptibility to reinjury [29]—and thus further reflex inhibition. This cyclical mechanism for ongoing pain is often referred to as the vicious cycle of CLBP. [30]

Disturbance of higher level information processing in the motor control system is believed to occur in CLBP as well, [30] including loss of discrete cortical organization of inputs to back muscles. [31] Even after apparent recovery from an individual episode of LBP, MCI of the LM can continue, leading to a higher risk of future episodes. [32]

Reversal of Motor Control Impairment Reduces Pain and Disability in CLBP

For rehabilitation to be effective, MCI needs to be overcome. Motor control exercises (i.e., exercises designed to improve the function of spine stabilizing musculature and the control of posture and movement, including exercises guided by ultrasound biofeedback) have been found to override the involuntary motor control system and help reverse impaired motor control [33], with subsequent reduction in pain and disability in CLBP.[34] In addition to reducing symptoms in CLBP, targeted training can reduce long-term recurrence of LBP and reduce the severity of recurrences that do occur.[25] Motor control exercises are frequently attempted in the physiotherapy clinic, but are not effective in all CLBP patients due to technical difficulty, challenges in teaching, implementation and patient compliance

Overriding Multifidus Muscle Inhibition with an Implanted Stimulator

A new approach to overcoming MCI in CLBP is the use of an implanted device to electrically stimulate the medial branch of the dorsal ramus nerve and cause the LM to contract episodically, thereby overriding the reflex inhibition. Electrical stimulation has already been shown to restore voluntary activation to quadriceps muscles chronically inhibited by MCI secondary to knee injury, with improvements in muscle strength and functional performance. [35, 36] From an anatomical and physiological point of view the ideal target for stimulation in CLBP are the deep LM fascicles across the area of pain [37] which are inaccessible from surface electrical stimulation.

The aim of this feasibility study was to test the hypothesis that, in patients with CLBP, electrical stimulation of the medial branch of the dorsal ramus nerve to contract the multifidus can improve the severity of CLBP and its impact on disability and quality of life.

Materials and methods

Patients

Patients were recruited between June 2011 and October 2012 at 4 sites in Belgium and the UK. Local institutional ethics committees approved the feasibility study and all patients were enrolled after written informed consent was obtained. The study was conducted in accordance with local regulations and ISO 14155.

Inclusion criteria included chronic non-specific low back pain (>90 days at time of enrolment); 18–60 years of age; Oswestry Dis- ability Index >25 (on 100-point scale) despite physical therapy and medical management; compromised neural drive to the LM on a prone Weighted Upper Extremity Lift Test (WUELT) [16] as deter- mined by a change in thickness of <20% of the LM during contraction on the right or left side at L4 or L5. The WUELT is an assessment of the change in thickness of the LM when a prone patient lifts a small weight with an upper extremity abducted to 120 degrees.

Exclusion criteria included previous back surgery or present indication for back surgery; previous interventional pain procedure(s) (including medial branch rhizotomy) that could affect the contraction of the LM in response to electrical stimulation; body mass index >35; currently implanted active implantable device(s); potential secondary gain; inability or unwillingness to comply with study protocol.

None of the patients were considered by the investigators to be eligible for Spinal Cord Stimulation or other neuromodulation therapies.

Study Design

The design was a prospective, multicenter, open-label single arm study aiming to characterize the performance of electrical stimulation to elicit episodic multifidus muscle contraction as a treatment for CLBP. Enrolled patients completed a medical history, physical examination and baseline clinical assessments including a low back pain Visual Analog Scale (VAS), Oswestry Disability Index (ODI), EQ-5D-3L assessment of quality of life, medication inventory, work status and WUELT.

Patients were implanted with a commercially available neurostimulator, including leads and implantable pulse generator (IPG), selected at the discretion of the investigator. Stimulation threshold testing and programming of the device occurred at the Therapy Activation Visit within 14 days of implant, and patients were instructed to deliver stimulation in two sessions of 20 min each day. At the four-month post-Activation Visit, therapy was withdrawn by collecting the external controllers such that patients could not deliver stimulation. At the five-month post-Activation Visit the external controllers were returned and patients were told to self- deliver treatment as needed (PRN) up to two 20-min sessions daily. Patients continued to be monitored quarterly through the final study visit at two years. Endpoint data were collected at Baseline, Implant, Activation, and at one, two, three, and five months post-Activation.

Patients were permitted to continue medication as well as adjust medications as needed during the study. All medication usage was recorded in a diary through three months. Patients also were per- mitted to continue previous participation in exercise. No other treatments targeted at LBP were permitted, including non-prescription medications, devices, adjunctive modalities (e.g., physical therapy, chiropractic) or interventional procedures, unless agreed to by the investigator. No exercise program was prescribed as part of the ongoing treatment.

Implant Procedure

The physician selected commercially available neurostimulation systems. The leads were placed under fluoroscopy at the edge between the transverse process and the superior articular process of L3 such that the distal electrodes were close to the medial branch of the dorsal ramus of the spinal nerve as it crosses the L3 transverse process (Fig. 2). The position of the needle for delivery of the leads was similar to needle placement for medial branch rhizotomy. Per- forming a 2 Hz twitch threshold test and observing and palpating the resulting multifidus contractions at outputs well above thresh- old verified lead position. A lead position was accepted if twitch thresholds were below 1 V or 1 mA and contractions were strong at an output of less than 2 mA or 2 V at 210μs pulse width.

The leads were attached to muscular fascia with the tapered distal end of the suture sleeve (anchor) partially inserted into the muscle. Pocket creation for the IPG and tunneling of the leads was similar to the procedure routinely used for spinal cord stimulation. Depending on each site's routine practice, patients were discharged either on the same day or within a day or two of surgery.

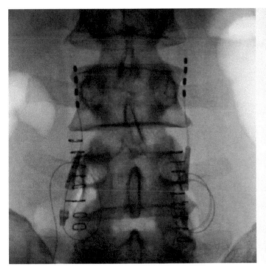
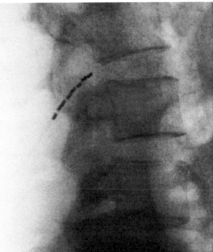

Figure 2: Fluoroscopic images of implanted leads.

Patients were instructed to avoid large or abrupt movements to minimize the risk of lead migration during the first 30 days following implant. Suspected lead migration or fracture (e.g., marked increase in impedance or sudden cessation of sensation of muscle contraction) were confirmed by comparing x-ray images of current lead position to fluoroscopic images of lead position at time of implant.

Programming

Stimulation threshold and impedance measurements were per- formed at time of implant and at each of the follow-up visits. All patients had the stimulation frequency set to 20 Hz and pulse width to 210 μsec which elicits smooth contraction of the LM. Stimulation amplitude was programmed to approximately 80% of the operating range (i.e., at the 80% point between twitch threshold and tolerance threshold) and several stimulation cycles were tested at this setting. Final output settings were fine-tuned upward if the patient felt the need for a stronger contraction or downward if the test cycles were perceived as uncomfortable.

During treatment, stimulation cycled between a 10-sec pulse train at 20 Hz (i.e., muscle contraction) followed by 20 sec of no stimulation (i.e., muscle relaxation) to avoid muscle fatigue. Stimulation amplitude ramped up and down slowly to avoid a "startle effect" due to sudden contraction onset or release.

Stimulation Delivery

From the Activation Visit until the four-month follow-up, each patient self-administered two 20-min stimulation sessions per day, one in the morning and one in the evening (ideally around the same time every day). During the sessions, the patients lay prone with a pillow under the lower abdomen or hips to ensure the LM was relaxed. To initiate stimulation patients used their external controller to activate the programmed sequence in the IPG. The external controller could be used to interrupt or discontinue stimulation at any time.

Data Management and Analysis

Data were recorded on electronic Case Report Forms by site staff. Data quality and compliance with protocol and regulatory requirements were assessed at regular monitoring visits by an external CRO. The VAS, ODI and EQ-5D were analyzed using SASv9.3 (Cary, NC, USA). Outcomes were summarized with descriptive statistics and p-values were assessed with a two-sided, paired t-test on the change from baseline. Data are summarized for the on-therapy three-month post-activation visit and the five-month post-activation visit following one month of therapy withdrawal.

Other outcomes included stimulation threshold, stimulation amplitude, impedance and use of medication for back pain. These outcomes were analyzed with descriptive statistics. All continuous outcomes are presented as mean ± standard deviation.

Safety was assessed as the cumulative frequency of adverse events related to the device and/or implant procedure from time of implant.

Results

Patient Demographics

Of the 28 patients enrolled, 26 patients were implanted with a stimulator and leads (mean duration of surgical procedure 105 ± 39 min). All patients had chronic LBP, mean duration 6.2 years (range 1.2–29.6) with 42.3% of patients experiencing bilateral and 57.7% experiencing unilateral LBP. Table 1 summarizes the demographics of the implanted patients. Seven patients withdrew between device implantation and the three-month endpoint: five due to lead migrations, one due to infection which led to device removal, and one after treatment was suspended pending recovery from unrelated surgery (Fig. 3). The efficacy cohort consists of the 19 patients who reached the three-month endpoint (Table 2). The safety analysis (N = includes all patients in whom an implant was attempted.

Pain (VAS)

At baseline, the average LBP VAS was 67.3 ± 11.1 mm (100 mm scale) (Fig. 4). At the three-month endpoint, the average LBP VAS had dropped to 40.8 ± 23.8 mm, a statistically significant improvement of 26.4 ± 22.3 mm or 39.7 ± 33.4% (p ≤ 0.0001). At three months, 14 out of 19 patients (73.7%) reported a minimally important change (MIC) of either ≥15 mm or ≥30% [38] on the LBP VAS

Table 1. Patient Demographics at Baseline.

Male, N (%)	10 (38.5)
Female, N (%)	16 (61.5)
Age, years—mean (min, max)	43.9 (23, 59)
Duration of back pain, years—mean (min, max)	6.2 (1.2, 29.6)
Body mass index, mean (min, max)	27.6 (19.1, 34.8)
<25, N (%)	7 (26.9)
25–30, N (%)	10 (38.5)
30–35, N (%)	9 (34.6)
Predominant pain, N (%)	
Unilateral	15 (57.7)
Bilateral	11 (42.3)
Work status, N (%)	
Full time	4 (15.4)
Part time	1 (3.8)
Disability leave	15 (57.7)
None or other	6 (23.1)

Disability (ODI)

The ODI score decreased from 38.5 ± 14.6 at baseline to 27.6 ± 15.6 at the three-month endpoint, representing a statistically significant average improvement of 10.9 ± 9.6 (p = 0.0001) or 29.6 ± 29.3%. At three months, 12 out of 19 patients (63.2%) reported a MIC of either ≥10 points or ≥30% on the ODI.[39]

Five of the 11 patients (45%) on disability leave for their LBP at baseline had resumed work by three months.

Quality of Life (EQ-5D-3L)

The EQ-5D score increased from 0.43 ± 0.34 at baseline to 0.70 ± 0.21 at the three-month endpoint, representing a statistically significant average improvement of 0.27 ± 0.24 points (p = 0.0002). At three months, 16 out of 19 patients (84.2%) reported an increase in EQ-5D and none reported a decrease

Durability of Effect

Stimulation was temporarily suspended between months 4 and 5 to test durability of effect. The VAS reductions were maintained through this period with a statistically significant improvement over baseline of 27.6 ± 27.3 (p = 0.0005) or 39.1 ± 40.6% at month 5 (N = 18) with 66.7% of patients reporting a MIC in LBP VAS despite unmasked treatment withdrawal. Further, 50% of patients reported ≥50% reduction in LBP VAS.

ODI and EQ-5D scores at month 5 also showed a sustained improvement (n = 19). Average ODI improvement over baseline after the one-month therapy withdrawal was 12.1 ± 14.4 (p = 0.0017) or 31.6 ± 31.5% with 52.6% of patients reporting a MIC in ODI. The average EQ-5D improvement over baseline was 0.20 ± 0.43 (p = 0.06) with 52.6% of patients reporting an improvement in EQ-5D.

Chapter 7

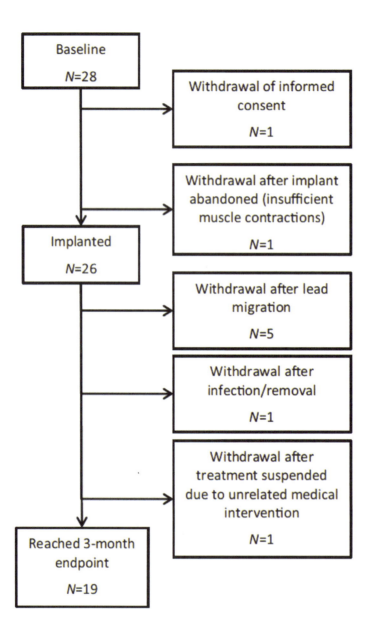

Figure 3: Patient accountability.

CLBP: restoration of dynamic stability

Table 2. Change in Efficacy Outcomes After Electrical Stimulation of the Lumbar Multifidus Compared With Baseline.

3-month endpoint Endpoint	N	Baseline, mean (SD)	Change vs. baseline, mean (SD)	p-value†	Response rate, % patients‡
VAS, mm	19	67.3 (11.1)	26.4 (22.3)	<0.0001	73.7 (14/19)
ODI	19	38.5 (14.6)	10.9 (9.6)	0.0001	63.2 (12/19)
EQ-5D	19	0.43 (0.34)	0.27 (0.24)	0.0002	
Post-off 5-month endpoint*					
VAS, mm	18	68.2 (10.6)	27.6 (27.3)	0.0005	66.7 (12/18)
ODI	19	38.5 (14.6)	12.1 (14.4)	0.0017	52.6 (10/19)
EQ-5D	19	0.43 (0.34)	0.20 (0.43)	0.06	

*Post-off data for the first three patients were collected at month 4 rather than month 5.
†Calculated using paired t-test.
‡Response criteria (minimal important change) was ≥30% or ≥15 mm for VAS and ≥30% or ≥10pts for ODI (not applicable to EQ-5D).
EQ-5D, EuroQol; ODI, Oswestry Disability Index; SD, standard deviation; VAS, visual analogue scale.

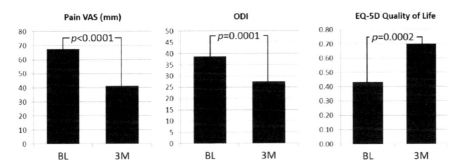

Figure 4: Change in efficacy outcomes at three months post-activation follow-up (N=19)

Medication Use

Of the 19 patients, 12 were on medication for LBP (including opioids, NSAIDs, anti-depressants, and sleep aids) at the time of the procedure and 7 were not. Of the 12 with pre-procedure medications, 8 either discontinued use or had decreases in the number and/or dose prior to the three-month endpoint. The remaining 4 with pre-procedure medications had no change in their medication for LBP at the three-month endpoint. Of those not on pre-procedure LBP medications, all remained off LBP medication at the three- month endpoint.

Stimulation Parameters

During stimulation, contraction of the multifidus could be felt by the patient and seen and palpated by the observer from approximately L1 to S1. The intensity and extent (number of levels) of con- traction differed between patients.

Since both voltage and current control devices were used, volt- ages have been converted to mA based on impedance measurements taken at that follow-up visit, thereby allowing aggregate data to be presented.

The average stimulation output required to produce smooth con- traction (stimulation threshold) at implant was 0.7 ± 0.7 mA (Table 3). After a post-implantation elevation in stimulation thresh- olds (average of 1.5 ± 1.9 mA at therapy initiation visit), thresholds stabilized at two months, with an average of 1.0–1.1 mA. Lead impedance averaged 967 ± 471 Ω at implant and stabilized to 550 ± 37 Ω at three months. The stimulation amplitude (i.e., amplitude used until the subsequent follow-up visit), was 2.6 ± 1.9 mA at therapy initiation and increased to 3.3 ± 1.9 mA at three months as a result of patient requests for stronger contractions at the one- and two-month follow-up visits.

Table 3. Stimulation Parameters Used for Electrical Stimulation of the Lumbar Multifidus (# of Patients = 19).

Follow-up	Implant	Therapy initiation	One month	Two months	Three months
Pulse width	210 or 212 µs (depending on the available settings of the IPG used). No change throughout the study				
Stimulation thresholds†					
	(N=23)	(N=29)	(N=33)	(N=33)	(N=30)
Amplitude (mA)	0.7±0.7	1.5±1.9	1.3±1.5	1.0±0.6	1.1±0.9
Lead impedance					
	(N=21)	(N=28)	(N=32)	(N=33)	(N=30)
Lead impedance (Ω)	967±471	486±181	537±199	566±220	550±202
Stimulation amplitude used for therapy delivery until next follow-up‡					
	(N=26)	(N=28)	(N=35)	(N=35)	(N=35)
Amplitude (mA)	NA	2.6±1.9	3.1±2.0	3.3±2.0	3.3±1.9

†The minimum amplitude required to produce smooth contraction.
‡That is, the amplitude of stimulation as programmed into the implantable pulse generator at the conclusion of the follow-up visit.
All results are ± standard deviation; N, number of leads for which the data are available; NA, not applicable.
NB. The number of leads for which data are available varies because (a) the implant procedure did not permit repeated measurements (required to collect stimulation thresholds), (b) in some of the earlier patients (as permitted by the protocol), unilateral stimulation was programmed and therefore only unilateral data recorded, and (c) threshold and impedance data is not available for leads affected by high impedance or migration.

Safety

In a safety population of 27 patients, a total of 97 adverse events (AEs) were reported, 37 of which were unrelated to the device or procedure.

Table 4. Device- and/or Procedure-Related Adverse Events.

	No. events	No. patients	% patients	Related to procedure	Related to device	Required surgery
Abnormal healing	1	1	3.7	1	0	0
Anaesthesia complications	0	0	0.0	1	0	0
Fever	1	1	3.7	0	1	0
Inadequate stimulation						
Not otherwise specified	1	1	3.7	0	1	0
Lead migration	9	8	29.6	4	9	0
High impedance	2	2	7.4	1	2	0
IPG malfunction	2	2	7.4	0	2	0
Infection	1	1	3.7	2	0	1
Musculoskeletal stiffness	2	2	7.4	2	0	0
Nervous system irritation/injury	2	1	3.7	2	0	0
Overstimulation of tissue	5	3	11.1	0	5	0
Pain	8	4	14.8	3	5	0
Risks associated with any surgical procedure, regardless of type	1	1	3.7	1	0	0
Seroma	1	1	3.7	1	0	0
Surgical intervention for device issue***						
Discomfort due to lead anchor	2	2	7.4	1	2	2
Lead migration	12	10	37.0	11	12	12
High impedance	2	2	7.4	1	2	2
IPG migration	2	2	7.4	2	2	2
IPG failure	1	1	3.7	0	1	1
Tissue injury	1	1	3.7	0	1	0
Undesired sensations						
Non-target area	1	1	3.7	0	1	0
Target area	1	1	3.7	0	1	0
All events	58	20	74.1	33	47	20

***Surgical intervention for infection captured separately.

Device and/or Procedure Related

Sixty device and/or procedure related AEs occurred in 20 patients (74%) (Table 4). Of these, 27 were device related, 13 were procedure related, and 20 were both device and procedure related. The most frequent AEs included lead migration leading to surgical intervention or inadequate stimulation (21 events), pain (8 events) and overstimulation of tissue (5 events). Twenty of the 60 related AEs resulted in a surgical procedure to address the event (all device revisions or explants). Two device and/or procedure related SAEs were reported: one nausea/vomiting due to surgical anesthesia, and one infection leading to device explant.

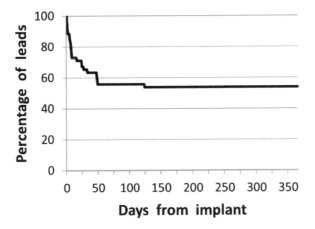

Figure 5: Number of days till primary (first) lead migration events reported.

Lead Migration

Sequelae of lead migration, including inadequate stimulation and surgical revision, were the most commonly reported device and/or procedure related AEs, with a total of 21 events that accounted for 12 of the 20 reasons for additional surgery. Of the 13 patients that experienced at least one lead migration, five had ≥2 migrations, two had ≥3 migrations and one experienced 4 migrations. Of the 12 surgeries performed to address lead migration, 11 were revision procedures to restore the ability to contract the multifidus and 1 was an explant. In all cases, surgery to address lead migration was performed solely if the patient wanted to have the lead repositioned. The majority of the migrations occurred shortly after implant (Fig. 5), with only 73% of primary lead implants remaining in place after 10 days and only 54% remaining in place at four months. Six of the patients who experienced lead migration withdrew from the study prior to the three month endpoint, although only 5 of those withdrawals were due to lead migration. Seven of the patients who experienced lead migration reached the three-month endpoint and are included in the efficacy analysis. Six of those seven had undergone lead revision prior to the three-month endpoint while one had continued with unilateral therapy following migration of the contralateral lead.

Discussion

Despite the multitude of treatments available to address LBP, for the 7% of patients that continue to suffer for longer than three months the chance of recovery is low.[40] We hypothesize that, for many patients, the reason for this is chronic inhibition of the lumbar multifidus, following an acute episode of LBP.[41] Without the coordinated efforts of a normally functioning motor control system, the lumbar spine joints may move outside their pain-free zone, leading to re-injury, impaired function and CLBP. A prospective, open label feasibility study with an open label withdrawal phase was con- ducted to characterize the performance of electrical stimulation of the lumbar multifidus in treatment of CLBP. Episodic stimulation of the medial branch of the dorsal ramus at L3 to contract the multifidus resulted in statistically significant and clinically important improvements with the majority of patients experiencing a clinically important reduction in pain (73.7%) and disability (63.2%) as well as an improvement in quality of life (84.2%) at three months. A one- month therapy withdrawal phase demonstrated durability of the effect with the majority of patients continuing to experience a clinically significant reduction in pain (66.7%) and disability (52.6%) as well as an improvement in quality of life (52.6%) at five months.

Research has shown that specific exercises to restore control to key spine stabilizing muscles, including the multifidus, can result in

improvement in the severity of symptoms of LBP, as well as a reduction in recurrence. [25] However, researchers report that many people find it difficult to voluntarily contract their multifidus. [42, 43] Ultrasound imaging biofeedback has been proposed to facilitate patient training, but this technique is not commonly used [44] because it is difficult [45], expensive [44], and impractical. [42] Effective treatment of LBP by specific exercises also depends on a patient's dedication to a demanding, technically challenging, regular exercise program, and compliance can be a problem. Further, results can be disappointing and a new approach is needed. [46] The results of this study extend the work on treating LBP with specific exercises targeted at the multifidus and suggest that electrical stimulation may be a means of overcoming the obstacles previously identified with using exercises to restore control to the multifidus.

The safety profile was similar to that seen with peripheral nerve stimulation devices with the exception of a higher than anticipated rate of lead migration. The leads utilized in the study were commercially available neurostimulation leads that were anchored using suture sleeves attached to the muscular fascia. Thirteen of the 27 patients in whom an implant was attempted experienced at least one lead migration, with 21 lead migration events in all and as many as 4 events in a single patient. This high rate suggests commercially available neurostimulation leads should not be used for this application.

On average, patients maintained their improvements in their scores on the VAS, ODI and EQ-5D when stimulation was temporarily withdrawn for one month following four months of treatment, though there was a modest worsening of responder rates. This should be viewed in the context of other neurostimulation devices used for pain which exhibit substantial reversals of pain relief with therapy withdrawal. [47]

Most patients elected to resume regular use of their device after the month 5 visit. Reasons given for their decision included (1) the perception that it would help prevent recurrence, (2) to treat recurrences when they did occur (with anecdotal reports of relief subsequent to use), (3) to help them "get going in the morning," and (4) to create the pleasant sensation of having worked out the muscles. The patients' actions in using the device voluntarily in long-term follow-up suggest there may be a continuing benefit from ongoing stimulation.

There were several limitations to this study. The study was limited by the absence of a control arm. The numerous withdrawals secondary to lead migration further reduced the small sample size and may have resulted in an overestimation of efficacy if the withdrawn subjects were experiencing less efficacy than those that remained in the study. Compliance with therapy was recorded via a diary, and is therefore subject to error as the devices were unable to log usage. Pain medications were not kept constant, and therefore the pain reduction effect of stimulation may be underestimated. Data presented were limited to short term follow-up and did not include a Global Perceived Effect scale to assess patient satisfaction. There was heterogeneity in the specifics of implementation of the therapy including unilateral vs. bilateral stimulation and the specific model of IPG and leads implanted. The WUELT assessment was included as an endpoint but experience during the study revealed a number of limitations regarding the WUELT's validity in the setting of a multi- center trial. These limitations included high intra-operator and inter-operator variability in ultrasound naïve investigators, and dependency of muscle thickness changes on patient lifting techniques with some patients "cheating" due to fatigue thereby invalidating the results. Hence the WUELT data were not analyzed. Lastly, the lead migrations may have negatively impacted the efficacy assessments, for example, VAS, ODI and QoL, due to both the morbidity of surgery to reposition the lead, as well as the decreased cumulative exposure to stimulation due to those periods when one or both leads were not in the correct position. As a result of the small sample size there is uncertainty with regards to the validity of the conclusions drawn from the study. Further, it is unknown whether the improvements observed in pain, disability and Quality of Life would be sustained in long-term follow-up. Lastly, without a control arm it is difficult to determine the contribution of the placebo effect to the treatment response, although the modest reductions in efficacy observed during the open label withdrawal phase suggest that the contribution of the placebo effect may have been limited.

Conclusions

This feasibility study suggests that, in patients with CLBP, episodic contraction of the multifidus elicited by stimulation of the medial branch of the dorsal ramus with an implantable electrical stimulator decreases back pain and disability and increases quality of life. However, given the multiple limitations of the study, the results must be considered preliminary and a placebo effect cannot be ruled out. A lead design specific to this application is essential to reduce the incidence of lead migration.

References

1. Airaksinen O, Brox JI, Cedraschi C, et al. Chapter 4. European guidelines for the management of chronic nonspecific low back pain. *Eur Spine J*. 2006;15 Suppl 2:S192-300.
2. Gore M, Sadosky A, Stacey BR, Tai KS, Leslie D. The burden of chronic low back pain: clinical comorbidities, treatment patterns, and health care costs in usual care settings. *Spine (Phila Pa 1976)*. 2012;37:E668-677.
3. Wenig CM, Schmidt CO, Kohlmann T, Schweikert B. Costs of back pain in Germany. *Eur J Pain*. 2009;13:280-286.
4. Chou R, Deyo RA, Jarvik JG. Appropriate use of lumbar imaging for evaluation of low back pain. *Radiol Clin North Am*. 2012;50:569-585.
5. Kim C, Ward S, Tomiya A, al. e. Microarchitecture studies of the human multifidus muscle reveal its unique design as a major dynamic stabilizer of the lumbar spine. *54th Annual Meeting of the Orthopaedic Research Society*. , Vol. 1616. Rosemont, Ilinois: Orthopedic Research Society; 2008.
6. Wilke HJ, Wolf S, Claes LE, Arand M, Wiesend A. Stability increase of the lumbar spine with different muscle groups. A biomechanical in vitro study. *Spine (Phila Pa 1976)*. 1995;20:192-198.
7. Rosatelli AL, Ravichandiran K, Agur AM. Three-dimensional study of the musculotendinous architecture of lumbar multifidus and its functional implications. *Clin Anat*. 2008;21:539-546.
8. MacDonald DA, Moseley GL, Hodges PW. The lumbar multifidus: does the evidence support clinical beliefs? *Man Ther*. 2006;11:254-263.
9. Macintosh JE, Valencia F, Bogduk N, Munro RR. The morphology of the human lumbar multifidus. *Clinical biomechanics*. 1986;1:196-204.
10. Palmieri RM, Weltman A, Edwards JE, et al. Pre-synaptic modulation of quadriceps arthrogenic muscle inhibition. *Knee Surg Sports Traumatol Arthrosc*. 2005;13:370-376.
11. Hopkins J, Ingersoll C. Arthrogenic muscle inhibition: a limiting factor in joint rehabilitation. . *J Sport Rehabil*. 2009;9.
12. Colloca CJ, Keller TS, Moore RJ, Gunzburg R, Harrison DE. Effects of disc degeneration on neurophysiological responses during dorsoventral mechanical excitation of the ovine lumbar spine. *J Electromyogr Kinesiol*. 2008;18:829-837.
13. Hodges P, Holm AK, Hansson T, Holm S. Rapid atrophy of the lumbar multifidus follows experimental disc or nerve root injury. *Spine (Phila Pa 1976)*. 2006;31:2926-2933.
14. Kiesel KB, Uhl T, Underwood FB, Nitz AJ. Rehabilitative ultrasound measurement of select trunk muscle activation during induced pain. *Man Ther*. 2008;13:132-138.
15. Dubois JD, Piche M, Cantin V, Descarreaux M. Effect of experimental low back pain on neuromuscular control of the trunk in healthy volunteers and patients with chronic low back pain. *J Electromyogr Kinesiol*. 2011;21:774-781.
16. Kiesel KB, Underwood FB, Mattacola CG, Nitz AJ, Malone TR. A comparison of select trunk muscle thickness change between subjects with low back pain classified in the treatment-based classification system and asymptomatic controls. *The Journal of orthopaedic and sports physical therapy*. 2007;37:596-607.
17. Danneels LA, Coorevits PL, Cools AM, et al. Differences in electromyographic activity in the multifidus muscle and the iliocostalis lumborum between healthy subjects and patients with sub-acute and chronic low back pain. *Eur Spine J*. 2002;11:13-19.
18. Wallwork TL, Stanton WR, Freke M, Hides JA. The effect of chronic low back pain on size and contraction of the lumbar multifidus muscle. *Man Ther*. 2009;14:496-500.
19. Kiesel KB, Uhl TL, Underwood FB, Rodd DW, Nitz AJ. Measurement of lumbar multifidus muscle contraction with rehabilitative ultrasound imaging. *Man Ther*. 2007;12:161-166.
20. Lee SW, Chan CK, Lam TS, et al. Relationship between low back pain and lumbar multifidus size at different postures. *Spine (Phila Pa 1976)*. 2006;31:2258-2262.
21. Beneck GJ, Kulig K. Multifidus atrophy is localized and bilateral in active persons with chronic unilateral low back pain. *Arch Phys Med Rehabil*. 2012;93:300-306.
22. Hu ZJ, He J, Zhao FD, Fang XQ, Zhou LN, Fan SW. An assessment of the intra- and inter-reliability of the lumbar paraspinal muscle parameters using CT scan and magnetic resonance imaging. *Spine (Phila Pa 1976)*. 2011;36:E868-874.
23. Hides JA, Stokes MJ, Saide M, Jull GA, Cooper DH. Evidence of lumbar multifidus muscle wasting ipsilateral to symptoms in patients with acute/subacute low back pain. *Spine (Phila Pa 1976)*. 1994;19:165-172.
24. O'Sullivan P. Diagnosis and classification of chronic low back pain disorders: maladaptive movement and motor control impairments as underlying mechanism. *Man Ther*. 2005;10:242-255.

25 Hides JA, Jull GA, Richardson CA. Long-term effects of specific stabilizing exercises for first-episode low back pain. *Spine (Phila Pa 1976)*. 2001;26:E243-248.

26 Hodges PW, Richardson CA. Inefficient muscular stabilization of the lumbar spine associated with low back pain. A motor control evaluation of transversus abdominis. *Spine (Phila Pa 1976)*. 1996;21:2640-2650.

27 Taimela S, Kankaanpaa M, Luoto S. The effect of lumbar fatigue on the ability to sense a change in lumbar position. A controlled study. *Spine (Phila Pa 1976)*. 1999;24:1322-1327.

28 Kankaanpaa M, Taimela S, Laaksonen D, Hanninen O, Airaksinen O. Back and hip extensor fatigability in chronic low back pain patients and controls. *Arch Phys Med Rehabil*. 1998;79:412-417.

29 Panjabi MM. Clinical spinal instability and low back pain. *J Electromyogr Kinesiol*. 2003;13:371-379.

30 Panjabi MM. A hypothesis of chronic back pain: ligament subfailure injuries lead to muscle control dysfunction. *Eur Spine J*. 2006;15:668-676.

31 Tsao H, Danneels LA, Hodges PW. ISSLS prize winner: Smudging the motor brain in young adults with recurrent low back pain. *Spine (Phila Pa 1976)*. 2011;36:1721-1727.

32 Hides JA, Richardson CA, Jull GA. Multifidus muscle recovery is not automatic after resolution of acute, first-episode low back pain. *Spine (Phila Pa 1976)*. 1996;21:2763-2769.

33 Tsao H, Druitt TR, Schollum TM, Hodges PW. Motor training of the lumbar paraspinal muscles induces immediate changes in motor coordination in patients with recurrent low back pain. *J Pain*. 2010;11:1120-1128.

34 Bystrom MG, Rasmussen-Barr E, Grooten WJ. Motor control exercises reduces pain and disability in chronic and recurrent low back pain: a meta-analysis. *Spine (Phila Pa 1976)*. 2013;38:E350-358.

35 Stevens JE, Mizner RL, Snyder-Mackler L. Neuromuscular electrical stimulation for quadriceps muscle strengthening after bilateral total knee arthroplasty: a case series. *The Journal of orthopaedic and sports physical therapy*. 2004;34:21-29.

36 Stevens-Lapsley JE, Balter JE, Wolfe P, Eckhoff DG, Kohrt WM. Early neuromuscular electrical stimulation to improve quadriceps muscle strength after total knee arthroplasty: a randomized controlled trial. *Phys Ther*. 2012;92:210-226.

37 Kim C, Gottschalk L, Eng C, Ward S, Lieber R. The multifidus muscle is the strongest stabilizer of the lumbar spine. . *Spine J*. 2007;7:76S.

38 Dworkin RH, Turk DC, Wyrwich KW, et al. Interpreting the clinical importance of treatment outcomes in chronic pain clinical trials: IMMPACT recommendations. *J Pain*. 2008;9:105-121.

39 Ostelo RW, Deyo RA, Stratford P, et al. Interpreting change scores for pain and functional status in low back pain: towards international consensus regarding minimal important change. *Spine (Phila Pa 1976)*. 2008;33:90-94.

40 Hall H, McIntosh G. Low back pain (chronic). *BMJ Clin Evid*. 2008;2008.

41 Freeman MD, Woodham MA, Woodham AW. The role of the lumbar multifidus in chronic low back pain: a review. *PM & R : the journal of injury, function, and rehabilitation*. 2010;2:142-146; quiz 141 p following 167.

42 Van K, Hides JA, Richardson CA. The use of real-time ultrasound imaging for biofeedback of lumbar multifidus muscle contraction in healthy subjects. *The Journal of orthopaedic and sports physical therapy*. 2006;36:920-925.

43 Herbert WJ, Heiss DG, Basso DM. Influence of feedback schedule in motor performance and learning of a lumbar multifidus muscle task using rehabilitative ultrasound imaging: a randomized clinical trial. *Phys Ther*. 2008;88:261-269.

44 Jedrzejczak A, Chipchase LS. The availability and usage frequency of real time ultrasound by physiotherapists in South Australia: an observational study. *Physiother Res Int*. 2008;13:231-240.

45 Stokes M, Rankin G, Newham DJ. Ultrasound imaging of lumbar multifidus muscle: normal reference ranges for measurements and practical guidance on the technique. *Man Ther*. 2005;10:116-126.

46 Deckers K, Adam A, Adam N, Rens A. Resolving Chronic Non-Specific Low Back Pain (CNSLBP) requires a new approach. *Neuromodulation*. 2013;16:e 176.

47 Liem L, Russo M, Huygen FJ, et al. A multicenter, prospective trial to assess the safety and performance of the spinal modulation dorsal root ganglion neurostimulator system in the treatment of chronic pain. *Neuromodulation*. 2013;16:471-482; discussion 482.

Chapter 8

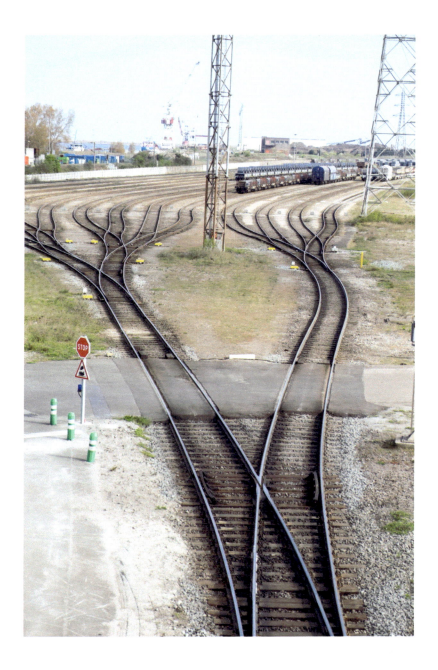

Chapter 8
General Discussion and Future Perspectives

History

The use of electric current to treat pain dates to the ancient Greeks who experienced numbness when standing in pools that contained electric fish. In modern medicine, electric current, of pre-specified frequency and amplitude is delivered to the spinal cord, the peripheral nerves, the motor cortex and the deep brain.

The first spinal cord stimulator for chronic pain was implanted by Norman Shealy in 1967, 50 years ago. [1] Steude et al. [2] report the stimulation of the Gasserian ganglion and Sweet[3] published the first experience with electrodes implanted along the peripheral nerve to control chronic pain. Since these first experiences the electrodes and pulse generators have been adapted to reduce the risk of complications. To increase the area covered with paresthesia, the basic principle of tonic spinal cord stimulation, multipolar electrodes and programmable stimulators have been developed.

In the 50 years since Shealy's publication, thousands of publications, textbooks, chapters, posters, oral presentations were dedicated to this subject. However, only 2 RCT's on tonic spinal cord stimulation were published. [4,5] The first study compared SCS with re-operation4 and the second was a comparison with conventional medical management.[5] Recently, the use of electrical current with an alternative waveform; the burst stimulation, the high frequency stimulation and the high density stimulation was introduced. The advantage of burst and high frequency stimulation is predominantly the fact that the paresthesia is not felt by the patient. Therefore, on theoretical grounds, a placebo/sham controlled study should be feasible. A randomized controlled trial compares BrustDR stimulation with tonic stimulation, the Sunburst® (T.Deer & al) study. The HF10 stimulation was also compared with tonic stimulation in the Senza® study. [6] Both studies were FDA designed non-inferiority RCT's. Performing placebo controlled studies, even with the new waveforms, faces several difficulties including ethical and psychological obstacles as is the case with most interventional pain management techniques that are reserved for patients who have already received a whole range of conventional and minimal invasive treatments. [7]

Spinal Cord Stimulation (SCS), even with the new waveforms such as High Frequency (10 KHz); BurstDR, and High Density, still struggles with some shortcomings and clinical outcome can be improved. A multicenter retrospective chart review to assess the duration of effect of SCS of 956 devices implanted between 2010 and 2013 with a follow-up time until mid-2016 (mean follow-up time of 2.23 years) (Van Buyten & al accepted for publication Neuromodulation) showed the highest explant rate for CRPS and low back pain, and higher explant rate for tonic rechargeable and HF10 rechargeable technology.

The dorsal root ganglion an ideal target for neurostimulation

Over the years, SCS has been studied in a variety of pain syndromes, the main challenge still is to find the correct lead placement to treat dermatome specific pain. Recently the research started to focus on stimulating another structure in the neuraxis, the dorsal root ganglion (DRG).

The DRG is sometimes called "The Gatekeeper", "The Highway intersection" and also "The Railway marshalling station" as it plays a key role in relaying sensory information to the central nervous system. The DRG plays a crucial role in the transduction and transmission of information from the periphery to the central nervous system (CNS), because it contains the greatest proportion of the body's sensory neurons. [8]

General discussion – Future Perspectives

Neuropathic pain, caused by injury of primary sensory neurons, is characterized by hypersensitivity due to a decreased threshold to action potential firing of nociceptors. The injury of the primary sensory neurons initiates the production of pro-inflammatory mediators released within the DRG.

The somatotopic arrangement of the DRG as such, and the effect on the somatosympathetic reflexes relays pain from different origin. Its localization in the neuraxis surrounded by dura mater but with very little CSF layer makes it an ideal structure to stimulate for neuropathic and sympathetically maintained pain.

The DRG has been the target of different interventional treatment options for the management of chronic pain, such as: ganglionectomy, and radiofrequency or pulsed radiofrequency current application adjacent to the DRG. The latter treatment involves the application of high frequency current to the DRG, the treatment is, however, of short duration, which is also reflected in the duration of effect.

Stimulation of the DRG has a direct cellular effect on the soma and other cellular structures of the primary sensory neurons, it has downstream effects on second order neuron in the spinal cord. It also acts at supraspinal regions sub serving higher order sensory functions and regions involved in cognitive and emotional processes involved in chronic pain.[9] It influences the peripheral anatomy, such as blood vessels. Basic research, using fMRI illustrated the effect of DRG stimulation of the brain reactivity to pain. (Hogan 2016 submitted)

The primary sensory neurons innervating somatic and visceral structures are housed in the DRG. Stimulation of these afferent neurons can produce a reflex arc involving interneurons that project to the inter-mediolateral cell column. Both spinal and supraspinal regions modulate this reflex which can induce potent and regional sympatholytic effects. The reduction in sympathetic outflow may result in peripheral vasodilation, vasculature and sympathetically associated pain mechanisms.[10]

Radicular back pain, due to disc herniation, compression and/or inflammation, potentially due to fibrosis after back surgery, of the DRG, is characterized by the radiation into the limbs according to a dermatomal distribution. Although SCS was demonstrated to be effective in the treatment of failed back surgery syndrome, the major problem remains finding the exact place for the lead to obtain paresthesia coverage of the painful area. Stimulation of the DRG was shown to overcome this problem and broadens the indication field because of the possibility to target the right level to stimulate.

Multicenter prospective trials show the beneficial effect of DRG stimulation on pain, QOL, functionality and mood status in patients with postsurgical neuropathic pain syndromes, CRPS, and radicular pain in FBSS patients.[11-14] A RCT shows statistically significant non-inferiority, even superiority of DRG stimulation versus tonic SCS in patients with CRPS for the primary outcomes.[15]

Because of the limited CSF layer surrounding the DRG and the position of the lead on the DRG in a narrow foramen, the accurate stimulation requires less energy compared to conventional SCS, which leads to a longer battery lifetime expectancy, thus reducing the cost of treatment. (chapter 6)

The downside of DRG stimulation are the technical difficulties in placing DRG stimulation leads. The technique consists in delivering a lead through a curved sheath and place the lead on the posterior part of the DRG through the epidural space into the intervertebral foramen. The positioning of the lead needs frequent AP/lateral fluoroscopic controls. The correct placement of the lead needs a learning curve. The placement of the leads in the high lumbar intervertebral foramina is easiest, low lumbar, thoracic and low cervical are the more difficult levels. One should be careful not to damage the DRG's in a narrow intervertebral foramen, careful preparation of the procedure by taking a preoperative CT scan to have an idea of the size of the targeted intervertebral foramen is a prerequisite.

Direct DRG stimulation has opened the door to new indications for neuromodulation. Many neuropathic pain conditions, impossible to treat with SCS can now be treated with a more specific, more targeted neurostimulation, with a known mechanism of action and supported by scientific evidence.

Stimulation of the Gasserian ganglion

The experience with stimulation of the Gasserian ganglion is older than the experience with DRG stimulation. This treatment has faced technical problems, such as inappropriate leads, lead migration and difficulties in reaching the correct target. We hypothesize that the Gasserian ganglion has the same function as the DRG in relaying the sensory information, but from the head and the face to the central nervous system allowing us to stimulate that structure to gate the propagation of painful stimuli from the periphery (V1, V2, V3). (chapter 2)

The introduction of the electrode requires a continuous fluoroscopic control, exposing the patient and the physician to a high dose of radiation. The electromagnetic neuro navigation technique allows with precision to reach the treatment target. We acquired the experience of using electromagnetic neuronavigation with the placement of the radiofrequency electrode in the Gasserian ganglion. The electrode placement is based on a previously taken CT-scan. During the procedure, the patients head is placed in a magnetic field. The reference points are ticked on the screen and on the patient's head. The computer matches the landmarks on the three-dimensional reconstruction and calculates the circle with a precision of 1 mm. Introduction of the electrode is followed real time on the navigation screen and only a short control of the position with a fluoroscopic image is required. This technique improves the safety and the precision of the electrode placement while reducing the radiation exposure. (chapter 4)[16]

Stimulation of the Gasserian ganglion is performed with electrodes designed for deep brain stimulation or electrodes used for spinal cord stimulation. These rather large electrodes are difficult to fixate and may cause damage to the surrounding tissue. We designed a tripolar, bent, tined electrode that was produced on demand by Medtronic (Model 09053). A retrospective analysis of 22 patients who have been implanted with such a custom-made electrode showed that the test stimulation was positive in 77.3% of the patients. Forty-four percent of them had a satisfactory pain relief at 24 months. The majority (82.4%) of these patients suffered from one or more complications, whith neck discomfort due to fibrotic tissue surrounding the connecting piece between the lead and extension being the most frequent complaint. We noticed a decline of the results over 24 months. These findings are now discussed with the lead manufacturer to improve the design of the electrode, so that complications can be avoided. [17] (chapter 3) Application of new wave forms, for instance irregular stimulation, of a known paradigm, such as burst stimulation, could enhance the long term effect and therefore prevent the decline in clinical effect, due to habituation. Clinical trials should be performed to confirm or refute this assumption.

Indirect stimulation of ganglia

C1C2C3 by stimulating the Occipital Nerve area.

Basic research and clinical evidence support the assumption that by stimulating the occipital nerve area we stimulate the trigemino-cervical complex, allowing us to treat many refractory headache conditions such as cervicogenic headache, chronic cluster headache, hemicrania continua, paroxysmal hemicrania, and other. An analysis of the long-term outcome of occipital nerve stimulation in patients with intractable chronic cluster headache showed that 19 out of the 51 patients included had additionally other types of headache. The success rate was slightly but not significantly higher in patients with cluster headache alone. After 3 years' follow-up, occipital nerve stimulation appeared to be still efficacious and safe.[18] Several other studies demonstrated the positive effect of ONS on cluster headache.[19]

This minimal invasive procedure is a rescue therapy for many of these patients who went through all other more conservative treatments (chapter 5)

Medial branch stimulation

Patients with chronic low back pain frequently experience a reflex dystrophy of the lumbar multifidus, which has a stabilizing role. The use of electrical stimulation of the quadriceps muscles that are chronically inhibited to restore the voluntary activation is already frequently used. A prospective, multicenter, open-label, single arm, feasibility on the use of an implanted device that electrically stimulates the medial branch of the dorsal ramus and cause the lumbar multifidus to contract episodically, thereby overriding the reflex inhibition was performed.[20] The leads were placed at the edge between the transverse process and the superior articular process of L3 such that the distal electrodes were close to the medial branch of the dorsal ramus of the spinal nerve as it crossed the L3 transverse process. During a 4-month period patients self-administered two 20-min stimulation sessions per day. The stimulation cycles between a 10-sec pulse train at 20 Hz followed by 20 sec of no stimulation. Twenty-six patients with chronic low back pain of mean duration of 6.2 years were implanted. Seven patients withdrew before the 3-month endpoint: 5 due to lead migration, 1 due to infection requiring device removal and 1 after treatment was suspended pending recovery from unrelated surgery. There was a significant reduction in pain, Oswestry Disability Index score and improvement in quality of life. The withdrawal of the therapy during 1 month had no negative impact on pain, disability and quality of life. At the 1 month follow-up visit patients already reported pain reduction, although restoration of the lumbar multifidus tonicity is not achieved.

These preliminary findings suggest that the stimulation of the medial branch of the dorsal ramus, also stimulates indirectly the DRG, because of the position of the leads very close to the DRG, and therefore also close to the sympathetic chain. This can explain the pain relief even before visible or measurable muscle restoration.

Further research to confirm these results is required. To overcome the problem of lead migration leads were adapted. A multicenter RCT is ongoing. (chapter 7)

Future perspectives, need for further research

The experience with DRG stimulation, Gasserian ganglion stimulation and occipital nerve stimulation give rise to the question: "Which ganglion do we stimulate?" and "How could the results be improved?"

Treatment of headache refractory to conservative management

Neurostimulation has progressively gained in interest for the treatment of different types of headache. The Gasserian ganglion is stimulated for the management of trigeminal neuropathy, occipital nerve stimulation was documented to be effective for the treatment of cluster headache, cervicogenic headache and migraine. However, not all patients report treatment success. The association of ONS with supraorbital and/or infraorbital nerve stimulation has been reported to provide pain relief in patients suffering migraine[21], different types of primary headaches[22], trigeminal neuralgia [23]

The phenotyping study of patients who received a permanently implanted device for ONS, learns that patients with migraine without aura and constant pain caused by compression, irritation or distortion of cranial nerves or upper cervical roots by structural lesions have a good chance for therapeutic success, while patients with medication overuse migraine have less favorable long-term outcome.[24]
The patient characteristics and diagnostic criteria to identify the patients with potentially higher successful outcome must be clarified.

Ganglion pterygopalatinum formerly sphenopalatinum

The ganglion pterygopalatinum has been targeted for the treatment of cluster headache on the basis of the close relation between headache and autonomic activation and the clinical observation of peripheral activation of the cranial autonomic systems with release of vasointestinal peptide and acetylcholine during the attack which may activate the trigeminal nociceptors.[25]

The pterygopalatine ganglion, formerly called the sphenopalatine ganglion, is considered to have a triangular, flatted form although there is still some uncertainty about the exact morphology of this ganglion. Some consider this ganglion polymorphic so it can take various forms like semi-lunar, rhomboidal, pear-shaped or fusiform with a length of 3-7mm. It is the biggest peripheral ganglion of the cranial parasympathetic system[26].

This ganglion is considered a parasympathetic ganglion since only pre-ganglionary parasympathetic axons synapse in this ganglion [27]. The pterygopalatine ganglion is considered the first relay station of the autonomic fibers after the fibers emerged from the pons. [28]

Stimulation of the pterygopalatine ganglion

Two studies report the use of pterygopalatine ganglion stimulation [29, 30]

The first study reports 6 patients with refractory cluster headache who were treated with electrical stimulation of the ganglion pterygopalatinum during an acute spontaneous or provoked attack.[29] The patients received a needle in the pterygopalatine fossa with a temporary single-contact stimulation electrode. Stimulation was delivered at varying frequencies, pulse widths and intensities. Eleven out of 18 attacks were completely resolved. The response was fast (1-3 min). The parameters that resulted in the best results were 50 Hz, pulse width 300 mcs and amplitude below 2 V.

In a well conducted randomized controlled trial Schoenen [30] included 32 patients who were implanted with an on-demand stimulator of the pterygopalatine ganglion, that can be activated by a hand-held stimulation device. When the patients felt the first signs of an attack they active the generator that was set to deliver ad random sham, sub perception of full therapy. Of the attacks treated with full stimulation 67.1% were relieved. In the sub perception-treated attacks 7.3% and in the sham treated 7.4 had a significant effect. Ten patients also experienced a reduction in attack frequency.

The stimulation of the pterygopalatine ganglion gives a dramatic effect within minutes of the start of stimulation but it also has a prophylactic effect on the occurrence of attacks.

Stimulation of the pterygopalatine ganglion was shown to have an abortive effect on cluster headache attacks. An experimental study showed that low frequency stimulation (5Hz) induced ipsilateral cluster headache attacks during or within 30 min following the stimulation. All these attacks were successfully treated with high frequency stimulation (80-120 Hz). These observations suggest that further research into the optimal stimulation frequency is warranted.

It must be clarified whether the prophylactic stimulation of the pterygoplatine ganglion also prevents the attacks.

Conclusions

Neurostimulation has longtime been reserved to the stimulation of the spinal cord. The stimulation of the Gasserian ganglion signed an era of further development and fine-tuning of the potential of neurostimulation. It is demonstrated that stimulation of the ganglia results in a more targeted effect, the DRG stimulation opened possibilities for the treatment of area's formerly inaccessible for stimulation.

It is important to note that indirect stimulation of the ganglia such as the trigemino cervical complex influences pain transmission. It seems that the stimulation of the medial branch of the dorsal ramus of the spinal nerve reduces pain and stimulates the lumbar multifidus, thus progressively restoring the muscle tonus.

There is an urgent need for further fine-tuning the optimal patient selection, and to develop adapted leads for each type of neurostimulation.

Chapter 8

References

1 Shealy CN, Taslitz N, Mortimer JT, Becker DP. Electrical inhibition of pain: experimental evaluation. *Anesth Analg.* 1967;46:299-305.
2 Steude U. Percutaneous electro stimulation of the trigeminal nerve in patients with atypical trigeminal neuralgia. *Neurochirurgia.* 1978;21:66-69.
3 Sweet WH. Control of pain by direct electrical stimulation of peripheral nerves. *Clin Neurosurg.* 1976;23:103-111.
4 North RB, Kidd DH, Farrokhi F, Piantadosi SA. Spinal cord stimulation versus repeated lumbosacral spine surgery for chronic pain: a randomized, controlled trial. *Neurosurgery.* 2005;56:98-106; discussion 106-107.
5 Kumar K, Taylor RS, Jacques L, et al. Spinal cord stimulation versus conventional medical management for neuropathic pain: a multicentre randomised controlled trial in patients with failed back surgery syndrome. *Pain.* 2007;132:179-188.
6 Kapural L, Yu C, Doust MW, et al. Novel 10-kHz High-frequency Therapy (HF10 Therapy) Is Superior to Traditional Low-frequency Spinal Cord Stimulation for the Treatment of Chronic Back and Leg Pain: The SENZA-RCT Randomized Controlled Trial. *Anesthesiology.* 2015;123:851-860.
7 Van Zundert J, Van Boxem K, Joosten EA, Kessels A. Clinical trials in interventional pain management: Optimizing chances for success? *Pain.* 2010;151:571-574.
8 Krames ES. The role of the dorsal root ganglion in the development of neuropathic pain. . *Pain Med.* 2014;15:1669-1685.
9 Koopmeiners AS, Mueller S, Kramer J, Hogan QH. Effect of electrical field stimulation on dorsal root ganglion neuronal function. *Neuromodulation.* 2013;16:304-311; discussion 310-301.
10 Loewy AD, Spyer KM. *Central regulation of autonomic functions.* New York - Oxford: Oxford University Press; 1990.
11 Liem L, Russo M, Huygen FJ, et al. A multicenter, prospective trial to assess the safety and performance of the spinal modulation dorsal root ganglion neurostimulator system in the treatment of chronic pain. *Neuromodulation.* 2013;16:471-482; discussion 482.
12 Liem L, Russo M, Huygen FJ, et al. One-year outcomes of spinal cord stimulation of the dorsal root ganglion in the treatment of chronic neuropathic pain. *Neuromodulation.* 2015;18:41-48; discussion 48-49.
13 Van Buyten JP, Smet I, Liem L, Russo M, Huygen F. Stimulation of dorsal root ganglia for the management of complex regional pain syndrome: a prospective case series. *Pain Pract.* 2015;15:208-216.
14 Schu S, Gulve A, ElDabe S, et al. Spinal cord stimulation of the dorsal root ganglion for groin pain-a retrospective review. *Pain Pract.* 2015;15:293-299.
15 Deer TR, Levy RM, Kramer J, et al. Dorsal root ganglion stimulation yielded higher treatment success rate for complex regional pain syndrome and causalgia at 3 and 12 months: a randomized comparative trial. *Pain.* 2017;158:669-681.
16 Van Buyten J, Smet I, Van de Kelft E. Electromagnetic Navigation Technology for More Precise Electrode Placement in the Foramen Ovale: A Technical Report *Neuromodulation.* 2009;12:244-249.
17 Kustermans L, Van Buyten JP, Smet I, Coucke W, Politis C. Stimulation of the Gasserian ganglion in the treatment of refractory trigeminal neuropathy. *J Craniomaxillofac Surg.* 2017;45:39-46.

18 Miller S, Watkins L, Matharu M. Treatment of intractable chronic cluster headache by occipital nerve stimulation: a cohort of 51 patients. *Eur J Neurol.* 2017;24:381-390.
19 Magis D, Jensen R, Schoenen J. Neurostimulation therapies for primary headache disorders: present and future. *Curr Opin Neurol.* 2012;25:269-276.
20 Deckers K, De Smedt K, van Buyten JP, et al. Chronic Low Back Pain: Restoration of Dynamic Stability. *Neuromodulation.* 2015;18:478-486; discussion 486.
21 Ellens DJ, Levy RM. Peripheral neuromodulation for migraine headache. *Prog Neurol Surg.* 2011;24:109-117.
22 Lambru G, Matharu MS. Peripheral neurostimulation in primary headaches. *Neurol Sci.* 2014;35 Suppl 1:77-81.
23 Shaparin N, Gritsenko K, Garcia-Roves DF, Shah U, Schultz T, DeLeon-Casasola O. Peripheral neuromodulation for the treatment of refractory trigeminal neuralgia. *Pain Res Manag.* 2015;20:63-66.
24 Paemeleire K, Van Buyten JP, Van Buynder M, et al. Phenotype of patients responsive to occipital nerve stimulation for refractory head pain. *Cephalalgia.* 2010;30:662-673.
25 Goadsby PJ, Edvinsson L. Human in vivo evidence for trigeminovascular activation in cluster headache. Neuropeptide changes and effects of acute attacks therapies. *Brain.* 1994;117 (Pt 3):427-434.
26 Siéssere S, Vitti M, Sousa LG, Semprini M, Iyomasa MM, Regalo SC. Anatomic variation of cranial parasympathetic ganglia. *Braz Oral Res.* 2008;22:101-105.

27   Windsor RE, Jahnke S. Sphenopalatine ganglion blockade: a review and proposed modification of the transnasal technique. *Pain Physician*. 2004;7:283-286.
28   Piagkou M, Demesticha T, Troupis T, et al. The pterygopalatine ganglion and its role in various pain syndromes: from anatomy to clinical practice. *Pain practice : the official journal of World Institute of Pain*. 2012;12:399-412.
29   Ansarinia M, Rezai A, Tepper SJ, et al. Electrical stimulation of sphenopalatine ganglion for acute treatment of cluster headaches. *Headache*. 2010;50:1164-1174.
30   Schoenen J, Jensen RH, Lanteri-Minet M, et al. Stimulation of the sphenopalatine ganglion (SPG) for cluster headache treatment. Pathway CH-1: a randomized, sham-controlled study. *Cephalalgia*. 2013;33:816-830.

Conclusions/Conclusies

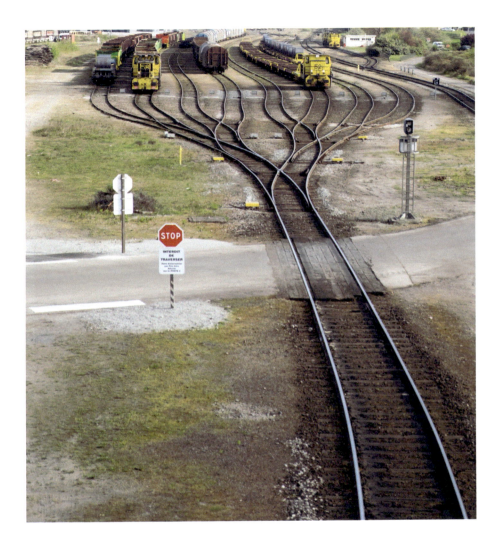

129

Chapter 9

Conclusions/Conclusies

Conclusion

Thanks to the technological evolution and to the possibility to stimulate electrically more specific anatomical structures, directly such as the Dorsal Root Ganglion, the Gasserian ganglion, the pterygopalatine ganglion or indirectly, the trigemino-cervical complex and the medial branch of the posterior ramus of the spinal ganglion, we have a shift of indications for neurostimulation from predominantly leg and back pain towards other indications such as cluster headache, migraine, trigeminal neuropathy and chronic non-specific low back pain.

Modern neuro-imaging technology and neuro-navigation techniques play an important role in the more targeted approach of neural structures for the treatment of chronic neuropathic pain syndromes, leading to better results.

Patients, physicians, researchers, health economists, health policy makers and health care related industry have a shared responsibility in controlling the global health care expenditure for the management of chronic pain syndromes. Research into the cost-effectiveness of these new techniques is of utmost importance

Conclusie

Dankzij de technologische evolutie en de mogelijkheid om meer specifiek anatomische structuren elektrisch te stimuleren, direct zoals het ganglion spinale (dorsal root ganglion), het ganglion van Gasser, het ganglion pterygopalatinum; of indirect, het trigemino-cervicale complex en de ramus medialis van de ramus posterior van de ganglion spinale, zijn de indicaties voor neurostimulatie veranderd van voornamelijk been- en rugpijn naar andere indicaties zoals cluster hoofdpijn, migraine, trigemus neuropathie en chronische niet-specifieke lage rugpijn.

De moderne neurologische beeldvormingstechnologie en de neuro navigatie technieken spelen een belangrijke rol bij de meer gerichte benadering van de neuronale structuren voor de behandeling van chronische neuropathische pijnsyndromen, en leiden zo tot betere resultaten.

Patiënten, artsen, onderzoekers, gezondheidseconomen, beleidsmakers van de gezondheidszorg en de gezondheid gerelateerde industrie hebben een gezamenlijke verantwoordelijkheid om het globale gezondheidsbudget voor de behandeling van chronische pijnsyndromen onder controle te houden. Het onderzoek naar de kosten effectiviteit van deze nieuwe technieken is van uitzonderlijk belang.

Curriculum vitae

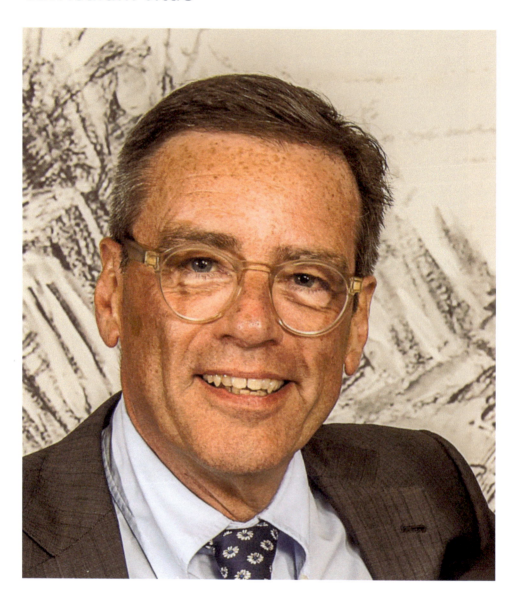

Jean-Pierre Van Buyten was born on the 9th of April 1954 in Sint-Niklaas Belgium, married to Carla Koslowski, is father of 2 daughters, Stéphanie and Barbara, and has three granddaughters, Noémie, Alixe and Jackie, and one grand sun Loic.

He followed secondary school in Sint Jozef Klein Seminarie in Sint-Niklaas. In 1972 he started medical school at the Universiteit Gent (UG) and further on the Vrije Universiteit Brussel (VUB) where he graduated in 1980 magna cum laude. His Anesthesia and Intensive Care residency started in 1980 consequently in Middelheim Hospital Antwerpen, Universitair Ziekenhuis Antwerpen in the department of Professor Dr. Guillaume Haenegreefs.

He started his career as an Anesthesiologist in 1984 in Algemeen Ziekenhuis Maria Middelares, currently AZ Nikolaas after merging with other hospitals. He was active as Anesthesiologist and Intensive Care Doctor during many years. Since his residency, he was more and more interested in the management of chronic pain. Currently he is the chairman of the Multidisciplinary Pain Center in the same hospital.

Dr. Van Buyten is the author of many scientific papers and gave number of lectures during international congresses on the treatment of chronic pain. Neuromodulation therapies are his main field of interest. Dr. Van Buyten is also actively involved in the board of many scientific societies and is currently the president of VAVP (Vlaamse Anesthesiologische Vereniging Voor Pijnbestrijding). He also serves in different advisory boards.

Apart from strictly medical activities he is involved in the board of the pension fund of Belgian caregivers (AMONIS) where he is currently vice president and president of the audit committee.

List of publications

Publications in peer reviewed journals

1   Carlier S, Van Buyten J. Spinal Cord Stimulation and Buerger's disease. The last resort therapeutic possibility ? *Belgian Journal of Medicine* 1990;46:1403-1407.

2   Belmans L, Van Buyten J, Adriaensen H. Accidental overdosing with intraspinal morphine caused by misprogrammation of a synchromed pump. A report of two cases. *Acta Anaesth Belg* 1997;48:93-97.

3   Adriaensen H, Maeyaert J, Van Buyten JP, Vanduynhoven E, Vermaut G, Vissers K. 2nd The Place of nerve blocks and invasive methods in pain therapy. *Best Pract Res Clin Anaesthesiol*. 1998;12:69-87.

4   Gybels J, Erdine S, Maeyaert J, et al. Neuromodulation of pain. A consensus statement prepared in Brussels 16-18 January 1998 by the following task force of the European Federation of IASP Chapters (EFIC). *Eur J Pain*. 1998;2:203-209.

5   Van Buyten J, Van Zundert J, Milbouw G. Treatment of failed back surgery syndrome patients with low back and leg pain: a pilot study of a new dual lead spinal cord stimulation system. *Neuromodulation*. 1999;2:258-265.

6   Van Buyten J. Tutorial II: Neuromodulation of Pain: Cost-effectiveness of Spinal Cord Stimulation *European Journal of Pain*. 1999;3.

7   Van Zundert J, Van Buyten JP. Current Use of Epidural Corticosteroids in Belgium: Results of a Recent Survey. *Pain Digest*. 1999;9:228-229.

8   Naumann C, Erdine S, Koulousakis A, Van Buyten JP, Schuchard M. Drug adverse events and system complications of intrathecal opioid delivery for pain: origins, detection, manifestations, and management. *Neuromodulation*. 1999:92-107.

9   Winkelmuller W, Burchiel K, Van Buyten JP. Intrathecal opioid therapy for pain: efficacy and outcomes. *Neuromodulation*. 1999;2:67-76.

10   Van Buyten J. Technique of Cervical Epidural Steroid injection. *Pain Digest*. 1999;9:228-229.

11   Abs R, Verhelst J, Maeyaert J, et al. Endocrine consequences of long-term intrathecal administration of opioids. *J Clin Endocrinol Metab*. 2000;85:2215-2222.

12   Van Buyten JP, Van Zundert J, Vueghs P, Vanduffel L. Efficacy of spinal cord stimulation: 10 years of experience in a pain centre in Belgium. *Eur J Pain*. 2001;5:299-307.

13   Everaert K, Devulder J, De Munck M, et al. The Pain Cycle: Implications for the diagnosis and treatment of Pelvic Pain Syndromes *Int Urogynecol J* 2001;12:9-14.

14   Maeyaert J, Buchser E, Van Buyten JP, Rainov NG, Becker R. Patient-controlled Analgesia in Intrathecal Therapy for Chronic Pain: Safety and Effective Operation of the Model 8831 Personal Therapy Manager with a Pre-implanted SynchroMed Infusion System. *Neuromodulation*. 2003;6:133-141.

15   Van Zundert J, Brabant S, Van de Kelft E, Vercruyssen A, Van Buyten JP. Pulsed radiofrequency treatment of the Gasserian ganglion in patients with idiopathic trigeminal neuralgia. *Pain*. 2003;104:449-452.

16   Van Buyten JP. The performance and safety of an implantable spinal cord stimulation system in patients with chronic pain: a 5-year study. *Neuromodulation*. 2003;6:79-87.

17   Van Zundert J, Brabant S, Van de Kelft E, Vercruyssen A, Van Buyten JP. Response to Zakrzewska's Letter to the Editor. *Pain*. 2004;109:520-522.

18   Taylor RS, Taylor RJ, Van Buyten JP, Buchser E, North R, Bayliss S. The cost effectiveness of spinal cord stimulation in the treatment of pain: a systematic review of the literature. *J Pain Symptom Manage*. 2004;27:370-378.

19   Van Buyten JP. Neurostimulation for chronic neuropathic back pain in failed back surgery syndrome. *J Pain Symptom Manage*. 2006;31:S25-29.

20   Van Buyten J. Spinal Cord Stimulation and Other Interventional Therapy Modalities for the treatment of Complex Regional Pain Syndrome. *Journal of Neuropathic Pain & Symptom Palliation* 2006;2:69-71.

21   Van Buyten JP, Lazorthes Y, Spincemaille GH. Prospective outcomes study on the Restore rechargeable neurostimulation system for neuropathic pain: A multi-center study. *Eur J Pain*. 2006;10:S 116.

22   De Andres J, Van Buyten JP. Neural modulation by stimulation. *Pain Pract*. 2006;6:39-45.

23   Kumar K, Buchser E, Linderoth B, Meglio M, Van Buyten JP. Avoiding Complications from spinal cord stimulation: Practical recommendations from an international panel of experts. *Neuromodulation*. 2007;10:24-33.

24   Van Buyten JP, Fowo S, Spincemaille GH, et al. The restore rechargeable, implantable neurostimulator: handling and clinical results of a multicenter study. *Clin J Pain*. 2008;24:325-334.

25   Van Buyten JP. Radiofrequency or neuromodulation treatment of chronic pain, when is it useful? . *European Journal of Pain* 2008;Suppl 2:57-66.

26   Van Buyten J, Smet I, Van de Kelft E. Electromagnetic Navigation Technology for More Precise Electrode Placement in the Foramen Ovale: A Technical Report *Neuromodulation*. 2009;12:244-249.

27   Van Buyten J, Linderoth B. "The Failed Back Surgery Syndrome": Definition and therapeutic algorithms: An Update. *Eur J of Pain Suppl*. 2010:273-286.

28   Paemeleire K, Van Buyten JP, Van Buynder M, et al. Phenotype of patients responsive to occipital nerve stimulation for refractory head pain. *Cephalalgia*. 2010;30:662-673.

29   Van Buyten JP, Hens C. Chronic stimulation of the Gasserian ganglion in patients with trigeminal neuropathy: A case series. *J of Neurosurgical review*. 2011;1:73-77.

30   Van Buyten JP, Linderoth B. Invasive neurostimulation in facial pain and headache syndromes. *European Journal of Pain Supplements*. 2011;5:409-421.

31   Alo K, Abramova M, Cantu F, et al. Technical update: Axial and radicular pain- recent advances in spinal pain mapping, epidural decompression and neurostimulation *Journal of Regional Anesthesia and Pain Medicine* 2011;37.

32   Van Buyten JP, Al-Kaisy A, Smet I, Palmisani S, Smith T. High-frequency spinal cord stimulation for the treatment of chronic back pain patients: results of a prospective multicenter European clinical study. *Neuromodulation*. 2013;16:59-65; discussion 65-56.

33   Al-Kaisy A, Van Buyten JP, Smet I, Palmisani S, Pang D, Smith T. Sustained Effectiveness of 10 kHz High-Frequency Spinal Cord Stimulation for Patients with Chronic Predominant Back Pain: 24-Month Results of the Prospective Multicenter European Study *Pain Medicine* 2014; 3: 347-354

34   Liem L, Russo M, Huygen FJ, et al. A multicenter, prospective trial to assess the safety and performance of the spinal modulation dorsal root ganglion neurostimulator system in the treatment of chronic pain. *Neuromodulation*. 2013;16:471-482; discussion 482.

35 Van Buyten JP, Smet I, Liem L, Russo M, Huygen F. Stimulation of dorsal root ganglia for the management of complex regional pain syndrome: a prospective case series. *Pain Pract*. 2015;15:208-216.

36 Kramer J, Liem L, Russo M, Smet I, Van Buyten JP, Huygen F. Lack of body positional effects on paresthesias when stimulating the dorsal root ganglion (DRG) in the treatment of chronic pain. *Neuromodulation*. 2015;18:50-57; discussion 57.

37 Liem L, Russo M, Huygen FJ, et al. One-year outcomes of spinal cord stimulation of the dorsal root ganglion in the treatment of chronic neuropathic pain. *Neuromodulation*. 2015;18:41-48; discussion 48-49.

38 Kustermans L, Van Buyten JP, Smet I, Coucke W, Politis C. Stimulation of the Gasserian ganglion in the treatment of refractory trigeminal neuropathy. *J Craniomaxillofac Surg*. 2017;45:39-46.

Book chapters

1   Van Buyten JP. Spinal cord stimulation. In: Szpalski M, Gunzburg R, eds. *Lumbar Spinal Stenosis*. Philadelphia: Lippencott Williams & Wilkins; 2000. 183-188.

2   Van Buyten JP. The use of radiofrequency and neuromodulation techniques. In: Szpalski M, Gunzburg R, eds. *The degenerative cervical spine*. Philadelphia: Lippencott Williams & Wilkins; 2001. 157-159.

3   van Dongen R, Van Buyten JP, van Kleef M. Speciële technieken: Ruggenmergstimulatie. In: Van Zundert J, Huygen F, Patijn J, van Kleef M, eds. *Praktische richtlijnen anesthesiologische pijnbestrijding, gebaseerd op klinische diagnosen*. Maastricht: NVA, VAVP, PKZ; 2009. 315-323.

4   Van Buyten JP. Interventional treatment for trigeminal neuralgia: radiofrequency and neuromodulation. In: Narouze S, ed. *Interventional management of head and facel pain: Nerve blocks and beyond*. New York: Springer; 2014. 59-64.

5   Van Buyten JP. Nouvelles modalités de neurostimulation. In: Lévêque M, ed. *Chirurgie de la douleur: de la lésion à la neuromodulation*: Springer; 2015.

6   Van Buyten JP. Traitement des douleurs faciales par stimulation des ganglions de Gasser et pterygopalatin. In: Lévêque M, ed. *Chirurgie de la douleur: de la lésion à la neuromodulation*: Springer; 2015.

7   Van Buyten JP. Neurostimulation for the management of Failed Back Surgery Syndrome (FBSS). In: Van de Kelft E, ed. *Surgery of the Spine and Spinal Cord. A neurosurgical focus*. Berlin: Springer Verlag; 10.1007/978-3-319-27613-7. 2016. 585-599.

Dankwoord / Acknowledgments

"It started with a kiss, never thought it would come to this..." zegt de song van Hot Chocolate, een discoband uit de jaren 70

De spreekwoordelijke "kiss" was een conversatie met Professor Maarten Moens op het jaarlijks congres van NANS (North American Neuromodulation Society) in Las Vegas december 2015, waar Maarten en ik moesten presenteren. Maarten overtuigde me ondanks mijn reeds gevorderde leeftijd om nog te beginnen aan een proefschrift voor het behalen van een doctoraat.

Mijn dankwoord gaat dan eerst en vooral naar Prof Dr. Maarten Moens, mijn promotor. Niet in het minst om zijn geloof in het feit dat een oudere collega die gans zijn carrière gewerkt heeft in een perifeer ziekenhuis ook bekwaam moet zijn om een proefschrift te schrijven.

Met een begeesterende Maarten Moens kan ik enkel maar goede herinneringen hebben aan deze periode waarin ik het privilege had om met jong talent te werken en goede discussies te kunnen hebben. Ik denk dat het uitzonderlijk is om een promotor te hebben die zo veel gaven tegelijk heeft en niet in het minst de humor, een van de meest waardevolle gaven.

Uiteraard is een proefschrift op mijn leeftijd een soort "retrospectieve", zoals je dat kan hebben van kunstenaars. In die zin werd ook de keuze van de co-promotores gemaakt, een moeilijke keuze uit collega's waarmee ik in de laatste jaren heb gewerkt en gepubliceerd. Natuurlijk speelde het onderwerp van het proefschrift een belangrijke rol in de keuze.

Professor Koen Paemeleire, neuroloog en wereldnaam in de kennis en de behandeling van hoofdpijn leerde ik kennen toen we samen een project hadden rond neurostimulatie en hoofdpijn, hij leerde me inzicht hebben in deze complexe pathologie en heeft me in de jaren die daarop volgden enorm geholpen in de juiste oriëntering en behandelen van patiënten met dergelijke problematiek, ik ben hem hiervoor enorm dankbaar.

Professor Frank Huygen, een gelijkgestemde van lange adem. Inderdaad neuromodulatie heeft lang niet op de prioriteitenlijst gestaan van onderzoeksprojecten in de academische wereld. Bij Professor Frank Huygen heb ik dit wel gevonden. De laatste jaren hebben we dan wel dikwijls de kans gehad om over dorsal root ganglion stimulatie te discussiëren, dank voor al deze boeiende gesprekken.

Dank ook aan de juryleden om de tijd te hebben genomen om dit proefschrift kritisch te bekijken, Prof. dr. Jan Lamote, Prof. dr. Ann Desmedt, Prof. dr. Maarten van Kleef, Prof. dr. Jacques Devulder.

Een speciaal dankwoord gaat naar Prof. Eric Cattrysse. Samen met Prof. Jan Clarijs hebben we nu reeds gedurende 22 jaar kadaver cursussen georganiseerd in het laboratorium van anatomie aan de Vrije Universiteit Brussel, en hebben we aan honderden collega's neuromodulatietechnieken kunnen aanleren, steeds samen met interessante lessen van anatomie.

Het ontwikkelen van het Pijncentrum in Sint-Niklaas had nooit gekund zonder de steun en de medewerking van de collega's van het eerste uur, Dr. Luc Vanduffel, Dr. Peter Vueghs, Dr. Iris Smet. Vandaag de dag is er nog steeds een aangename samenwerking met mijn rechtstreekse collega's, Iris Smet, Frank Thiessen, Franscesca Van der Puijl. Tezamen trachten we het enorme aanbod aan chronische pijn patiënten de baas te kunnen, en jonge collega's residenten op te leiden.

Ik zou ook in het bijzonder De Heren Koen Michiels, Afgevaardigd bestuurder van het AZ Nikolaas, en de Heer Erik Vlaeminck, investerings-en exploitatiemanager van het Medisch Departement AZ Nikolaas willen danken voor hun onvoorwaardelijke steun aan het Pijncentrum en hun geloof in onze projecten

Het werk eindigt niet als we het ziekenhuis verlaten. Samen met een handvol collega's uit het Vlaamse land hebben we de Flemish Pain Society gestart eind de tachtiger jaren. Luc De Colvenaer, Luc Vaduffel, Jan Maeyaert, Luc Jamaer, Marc Maes, stonden op de barricade om de belangen te verdedigen van een groepje specialisten die in navolging van de pioniers als Prof. Hugo Adriaenssens dit specialisme wouden ontwikkelen. Dit is dan mede dankzij de niet te stuiten energie, het onmetelijke enthousiasme, en de diplomatie van Prof. dr. Jan Van Zundert uitgegroeid tot de Vlaamse Anesthesiologische Vereniging voor Pijnbestrijding (VAVP) waarvan ik gedurende de laatste 6 jaar voorzitter mocht zijn. Ook in de strijd voor een degelijke nomenclatuur speelde hij een cruciale rol.

Ik wil van de gelegenheid gebruik maken om al deze collega's te bedanken voor hun inzet en vriendschap.

Een zeer speciaal dankwoord gaat naar Mevrouw Nicole Van Den Hecke. Ik durf te zeggen dat er zonder Nicole van VAVP, en misschien zelfs van de Pijntherapie in toto niet veel van in huis was gekomen in België. Nicole heeft zich jarenlang ingezet met woord en daad voor onze vereniging. Zij heeft meerderen van ons begeleid bij het behalen van een doctoraat. Haar onuitputtelijke databank en kennis van de literatuur, haar bereidheid tot reviewen, haar strikte deadlines hebben mij zeker geholpen. Nicole zal nooit pijn hebben, ze heeft alle pijnartsen in binnen en buitenland tot vriend.

Ook heb ik inspiratie gekregen en een bredere kijk op de maatschappij en de organisatie van mijn dienst dankzij enkele nevenactiviteiten.

Bij Amonis, het Belgisch pensioenfonds voor zorgverstrekkers, leerde ik als beheerder het reilen en zeilen van een financiële instelling, skills die ik heb kunnen gebruiken in mijn praktijk, en die mijn netwerk hebben uitgebreid tot een andere wereld en een andere manier van denken. Dank aan alle collega's van Raad Van Bestuur en het directiecomité van Amonis OFP en bijzonder aan Dr. Herwig Van Dyck.

De weg naar finaal dit proefschrift is in mijn geval dus zeer lang geweest en het resultaat van een carrière van meer dan 30 jaar pijntherapie en klinisch onderzoek hoofdzakelijk in Neuromodulatie. Daarom ben ik zeker dat ik in mijn dankwoord mensen zal vergeten die op één of andere manier betrokken zijn geweest of hebben bijgedragen tot de realisatie van dit project, het waren er zo veel. Aan al die vergeten collega's vrienden en medewerkers, dank U wel.

Wat is een mens zonder zijn familie en zijn gezin.

Clichés zeggen dat er achter elke sterke man een nog sterkere vrouw staat, en Generaal Patton pleegde te zeggen: "The General's wife is the General's General". Beiden gelden voor mijn begrijpende en geduldige echtgenote Carla, die me reeds 39 jaar helpt, bijstaat en zeer dikwijls uren heeft gewacht om me laat 's avonds na een drukke dag en vergaderingen nog een warme maaltijd voor te schotelen en nog een babbeltje te doen om me een update te geven over het gezin. Een dikke en hartelijke dank-U-zoen hiervoor.

Ook natuurlijk dank aan mijn beauty's en schatten van dochters Stéphanie en Barbara. Ondanks mijn frequente afwezigheid heb ik altijd veel liefde van jullie ondervonden. Samen met jullie toffe mannen hebben jullie gezorgd voor, tot hiertoe, vier schatten van kleinkinderen die regelmatig zorgen voor de nodige ambiance ten huize Van Buyten.

Finaal zou ik willen stellen dat dit werk werd geschreven uit dank voor een tot hiertoe rijk gevulde carrière, en betekent hopelijk een nieuwe boost om met de opgedane ervaring en kennis nog enkele jaren te kunnen bijdragen aan de verdere ontwikkeling van de pijntherapie.